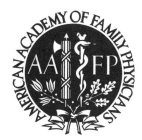

THE ACADEMY COLLECTION
Quick Reference Guides for Family Physicians

Gastrointestinal Problems

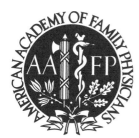

THE ACADEMY COLLECTION
Quick Reference Guides for Family Physicians

Gastrointestinal Problems

Edited by
MARTIN S. LIPSKY, M.D.
Professor and Chair
Department of Family Medicine
Northwestern University Medical School and
Evanston Northwestern Healthcare
Chicago, Illinois

With 10 Contributors

Series Medical Editor
RICHARD SADOVSKY, M.D., M.S.
Associate Professor of Family Medicine
State University of New York Health Science Center
Brooklyn, New York

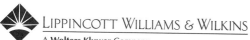

LIPPINCOTT WILLIAMS & WILKINS
A **Wolters Kluwer** Company

Philadelphia · Baltimore · New York · London
Buenos Aires · Hong Kong · Sydney · Tokyo

Acquisitions Editor: Richard Winters
Developmental Editor: Alexandra T. Anderson
Project Editor, AAFP: Leigh McKinney
Production Editor: Emily Lerman
Manufacturing Manager: Colin J. Warnock
Cover Designer: Mark Lerner
Compositor: Lippincott Williams & Wilkins Desktop Division
Printer: R.R. Donnelley–Crawfordsville

Library of Congress Cataloging-in-Publication Data
Gastroenterology / edited by Martin S. Lipsky ; with 10 contributors.
    p. ; c.m— (the Academy collection—quick reference guides for family physicians)
    Includes bibliographical references and index.
    ISBN 0-7817-2054-0 (alk. paper)
Gastroenterology—Handbooks, manuals, etc. 3. Family medicine—Handbooks,
manuals, etc. I. Lipsky Martin S. II. Series.
    [DNLM: 1. Gastrointestinal Diseases—diagnosis—Handbooks. 2. Gastrointestinal
Diseases—Therapy—Handbooks. WI 39 G2565 2000]
RC801 .G3762 2000
616.3′3—dc21
                                                                00-30963

Care has been taken to confirm the accuracy of the information presented and to describe generally accepted practices. However, the authors, editor, and publisher are not responsible for errors or omissions or for any consequences from application of the information in this book and make no warranty, expressed or implied, with respect to the currency, completeness, or accuracy of the contents of the publication. Application of this information in a particular situation remains the professional responsibility of the practitioner.

The authors, editor, and publisher have exerted every effort to ensure that drug selection and dosage set forth in this text are in accordance with current recommendations and practice at the time of publication. However, in view of ongoing research, changes in government regulations, and the constant flow of information relating to drug therapy and drug reactions, the reader is urged to check the package insert for each drug for any change in indications and dosage and for added warnings and precautions. This is particularly important when the recommended agent is a new or infrequently employed drug.

Some drugs and medical devices presented in this publication have Food and Drug Administration (FDA) clearance for limited use in restricted research settings. It is the responsibility of the health care provider to ascertain the FDA status of each drug or device planned for use in their clinical practice.

10 9 8 7 6 5 4 3 2 1

SERIES INTRODUCTION

Family practice is a unique clinical specialty encompassing a philosophy of care rather than a modality of care provided to a specific segment of the population. This philosophy of providing longitudinal care for persons of all ages in the complete context of their physical, emotional, and social environments was modeled by general practitioners, the parents of our modern specialty. To provide this kind of care, the family physician needs a broad knowledge base, appropriate evaluation tools, effective interventions, and patient education.

The knowledge base needed by a family physician is extraordinarily large. The American Academy of Family Physicians and other organizations provide clinical education through conferences and journals. Individual family physicians have written journal articles about a specific clinical topic or have tried to cover the broad knowledge base of family medicine in a single volume. The former are helpful, but may cover only a narrow segment of medicine, while the latter may not provide the depth needed to be useful in actual patient care.

The Academy Collection: Quick Reference Guides for Family Physicians is a series of books designed to assist family physicians with the broad knowledge base unique to our specialty. The books in this series have all been written by practicing family physicians who have special interest in the topics, and the chapters have been formatted to provide easy access to information needed at varying stages in the physician-patient encounter. Each volume is unique because each author has personalized the volume and provided a unique family physician perspective.

This series is not meant to be a final reference for the family physician who seeks a comprehensive text. The series also does not cover every topic that may be encountered by the family physician. The series does offer, in a depth determined appropriate by the authors, the information needed by the physician to handle the majority of patient encounters. The series also provides information to make patient care a combined doctor-patient effort. Specific patient education materials have been included where appropriate. Readers can contact the American Academy of Family Physicians Foundation for other resources.

The topics selected for *The Academy Collection* were chosen based on what family physicians said they needed. The first group of books covers office procedures, conditions of aging, and some of the most challenging diagnoses seen in family practice. Future books in the series will address skin conditions, occupational medicine, children's health, and women's health.

I welcome your comments. Please contact me at the American Academy of Family Physicians with your suggestions (Rick Sadovsky, M.D., Series Editor, The Academy Collection, c/o AAFP, 11400 Tomahawk Creek Parkway, Leawood, KS 66211-2672; e-mail: academycollection@aafp.org). This collection is meant to be useful to you and your patients.

Richard Sadovsky, M.D., M.S.
Series Editor

CONTENTS

CONTRIBUTING AUTHORS

Mari E. Egan, M.D.
Instructor of Family Medicine
Northwestern University Medical School
303 East Chicago Avenue, Morton 1-658
Chicago, Illinois 60611

Sanford R. Kimmel, M.D.
Associate Professor of Family Medicine
Medical College of Ohio
MCO Family Practice Center
1015 Garden Lake Parkway
Toledo, Ohio 43699-0008

Mitchell King, M.D.
Assistant Professor of Family Medicine
Northwestern University Medical School;
Department of Family Medicine
Glenbrook Hospital
2100 Pfingsten Road
Glenview, Illinois 60025

William B. Klein, M.D.
Resident in Family Practice
Medical College of Ohio and
St. Vincent Mercy Medical Center
Family Practice Residency
1015 Garden Lake Parkway
Toledo, Ohio 43614

Kurt Kurowski, M.D.
Assistant Professor of Family Medicine
Finch University of the Health Sciences/
Chicago Medical School
3333 Greenbay Road
North Chicago, Illinois 60064-3095

Martin S. Lipsky, M.D.
Professor and Chair of Family Medicine
Northwestern University Medical School and
Evanston Northwestern Healthcare
303 East Chicago Avenue, Morton 1-658
Chicago, Illinois 60611

Diane J. Madlon-Kay, M.D.
Associate Professor of Family Medicine
University of Minnesota
Minneapolis, Minnesota;
Family Medicine Residency Program
Regions Hospital
St. Paul, Minnesota 55101-2595

Jory A. Natkin, D.O.
Instructor of Family Medicine
Northwestern University Medical School;
Department of Family Medicine
Glenbrook Hospital
2100 Pfingsten Road
Glenview, Illinois 60025

Mark C. Potter, M.D.
Assistant Professor of Family Medicine
Loyola University Medical School
Maywood, Illinois;
Provident Hospital of Cook County
500 East 51st Street
Chicago, Illinois 60611

Arlene Sagan, M.D.
Clinical Instructor of Family Medicine
Northwestern University Medical School
ENH Medical Group
190 Waukegan Road
Deerfield, Illinois 60015

Robert M. Wolfe, M.D.
Instructor of Family Medicine
Northwestern University Medical School
303 East Chicago Avenue, Morton 1-658
Chicago, Illinois 60611

INTRODUCTION

....

Gastrointestinal symptoms are among the most frequent reasons for an office visit to a family physician. Virtually no office session passes without a busy family physician encountering at least one patient reporting nausea, diarrhea, abdominal pain, or one of a host of common gastrointestinal symptoms.

The goal of this book is to help physicians manage these symptoms. Chapters are organized by problems because most primary care encounters revolve around symptoms. Rarely do patients come in announcing their illnesses and requesting treatment.

The target audience for this book consists of practicing physicians. All the authors are family physicians who practice actively. This ensures that the material is relevant and useful to a family physician. Outpatient evaluation and management is the primary focus, although indications for hospital admission and more advanced treatment are outlined. Many tables and figures are presented to make the information readily accessible. Each chapter contains differential diagnoses and an approach for evaluating the patient directed by the history and physical exam. Laboratory work-up is provided along with suggestions for when a test or further evaluation is indicated.

In addition to being a quick office resource, the book also provides sufficient material for physicians who want to review gastroenterology or to brush up in preparation for recertification. Although this book is organized by symptom, all the major common gastrointestinal disorders are discussed, generally in the chapter of their most common presenting symptom. Medical students or residents who desire a straightforward review for examinations or who wish to treat patients more effectively should also find the content suitable to meet these needs.

I acknowledge the members of our family medicine department at Northwestern University Medical School and Evanston Northwestern Healthcare. In addition to contributing numerous chapters and meeting aggressive timelines, my colleagues at Northwestern provided critical review and made numerous beneficial suggestions. In particular, without the enthusiasm and help of Dr. Mitch King, I would not have attempted this project. Finally, Alexandra T. Anderson, our editor at Lippincott Williams & Wilkins, was instrumental to our book. Her insightful editing and sense of humor provided clarity and enthusiasm and made this an enjoyable project.

Martin S. Lipsky, M.D.

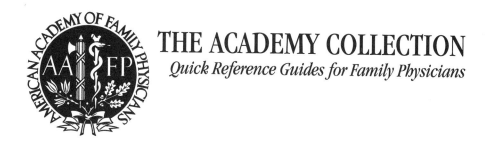

THE ACADEMY COLLECTION
Quick Reference Guides for Family Physicians

Gastrointestinal Problems

CHAPTER 1

Abdominal Pain in Adults

Mitchell King

DEFINITION

Abdominal pain is a common problem with a variety of presenting symptoms and potential causes. Diagnostic possibilities range from the chronic and benign (e.g, irritable bowel syndrome) to the acute and life-threatening (e.g., ruptured aortic aneurysm). Table 1.1 presents the most commonly diagnosed causes for abdominal pain seen by family physicians in the office setting.

CLINICAL MANIFESTATIONS

The mode of presentation determines the rapidity and setting for further evaluation. Initial triage of the patient involves determining the time course, location and severity of the pain, and the vital signs of the patient.

The Acute Abdomen

Patients with an "acute" abdomen typically are seen in emergency rooms, but on occasion may present to the physician's office. If the patient is hemodynamically unstable, then an abdominal aortic aneurysm (AAA) should be suspected. Acute abdominal pain presenting with a rigid abdomen and hemodynamic stability may be caused by perforation, infarction, or obstruction of an abdominal organ. These patients should undergo a limited evaluation and resuscitation before a physician proceeds with prompt operative intervention.

Localized Abdominal Pain

Localized abdominal pain (Table 1.2) can occur acutely, but generally in the outpatient setting the patient is hemodynamically stable and evaluation based on the history, physical examination, laboratory studies, and radiologic testing will uncover the cause.

   Epigastric pain may signify the presence of gastroesophageal reflux disease (Chapter 9), peptic ulcer disease (Chapter 9), biliary tract disease (Chapter 7), or pan-

---

T ABLE 1.1.   Possible causes of abdominal pain in the office setting

Acute gastroenteritis	Cholelithiasis
Urinary tract infection	Peptic ulcer disease
Irritable bowel syndrome	Urolithiasis
Pelvic inflammatory disease	Appendicitis
Gastroesophageal reflux disease	Ulcerative colitis
Diverticulosis	Muscular strain

T ABLE 1.2.   Differential diagnosis of abdominal pain by location

EPIGASTRIC
Gastroesophageal reflux disease
Peptic ulcer disease
Gastritis
Pancreatitis
Cholecystitis
Musculoskeletal
Cardiac (e.g., myocardial infarction/pericarditis)

RIGHT UPPER QUADRANT
Cholecystitis
Liver disease (e.g., hepatitis, cholangitis, abscess)
Gastritis
Peptic ulcer disease
Renal (e.g., stones, pyelonephritis)
Pulmonary (e.g., pneumonia, pleural disease, pulmonary embolus)
Musculoskeletal
Herpes zoster
Appendicitis
Subdiaphragmatic abscess

LEFT UPPER QUADRANT
Peptic ulcer disease
Gastritis
Splenic (e.g., splenomegaly, infarction, injury)
Pancreatitis
Abdominal aortic aneurysm
Cardiac (e.g., myocardial infarction, pericarditis)
Pulmonary (e.g., pneumonia, pleural disease, pulmonary embolus)
Musculoskeletal
Herpes zoster

RIGHT LOWER QUADRANT
Appendicitis
Mesenteric adenitis
Crohn's disease
Diverticular disease, including Meckel's diverticulum
Cholecystitis/biliary tract
Musculoskeletal
Pancreatitis
Herpes zoster
Gynecologic (e.g., pelvic inflammatory disease, ectopic pregnancy, endometriosis)
Renal (e.g., stones, infection)

continued

TABLE 1.2 *continued.* Differential diagnosis of abdominal pain by location

LEFT LOWER QUADRANT
Diverticular disease
Colitis
Crohn's disease
Bowel obstruction
Colon cancer
Musuloskeletal
Renal (e.g., stones, infection)
Gynecologic (e.g., pelvic inflammatory disease, ectopic pregnancy, endometriosis)
Herpes zoster

creatitis. Pain with pancreatitis, often referred to the back, is associated with nausea, vomiting, and possibly fever. Other potential causes of epigastric abdominal pain include those referred from the heart (myocardial infarction, pericarditis) or musculoskeletal system (costochondritis).

The **right upper quadrant** is the classic location for the pain of cholecystitis. Patients may also have nausea, emesis, and pain referral to the scapular region. The classic physical examination finding of a Murphy's sign is supportive. Murphy's sign is elicited by having the patient inspire during palpation of the right upper quadrant, in the region of the gallbladder. This sign is considered present when the patient experiences pain and abruptly halts inspiratory effort. Pain from nephrolithiasis can also occur in the right upper quadrant; typically, it is colicky and radiates to the back and groin. Right upper quadrant pain can occur with pyelonephritis, in which case back pain, dysuria, fever, and costovertebral angle tenderness typically are also present. Peptic ulcer disease and, less commonly, appendicitis can present with right upper quadrant pain. In addition, cardiac, pulmonary, and musculoskeletal causes must be considered in evaluating upper-quadrant abdominal pain.

Left upper quadrant pain occurs less commonly. Potential causes for left upper quadrant pain include peptic ulcer disease, pancreatitis, and splenic infarction. Pain from an AAA, as well as pulmonary, cardiac, and musculoskeletal sources, can also occur in the left upper quadrant.

The **right lower quadrant** is the classic location for pain from appendicitis. Appendicitis can initially occur with periumbilical pain that subsequently localizes to the right lower quadrant. This pain may be associated with fever and nausea/emesis that follow the onset of pain. Mesenteric adenitis can present with similar symptoms and can be difficult to distinguish from appendicitis. Crohn's disease, diverticulitis, ureterolithiasis, AAA, and musculoskeletal pain (e.g., rectal sheath hematoma) can also occur in the right lower quadrant. Less commonly, biliary tract disease and Meckel's diverticulum may be responsible for the patient's pain. In women, gynecologic causes (e.g., pelvic inflammatory disease, ectopic pregnancy, endometriosis, and ovarian torsion) must be considered.

The **left lower quadrant** is the classic location for pain from diverticulitis. Associated symptoms may include low-grade fever, anorexia, and nausea. Severe pain can signify the presence of a diverticular abscess. Although diverticulitis can occur in the right colon, in which case it may be indistinguishable from appendicitis, the usual location is the sigmoid colon. Left lower quadrant pain can also emanate from colitis (Chapter 13), Crohn's disease, colon cancer, bowel obstruction (e.g., adhesions, cancer), or AAA, or result from urologic, gynecologic, or musculoskeletal disease.

Chronic Abdominal Pain

Irritable bowel syndrome and peptic ulcer disease are the most common causes of chronic abdominal pain in patients who present to the family physician's office. Inflammatory bowel disease and diverticular disease also commonly cause chronic abdominal pain. Other potential causes include chronic pancreatitis, gastric cancer, and metabolic diseases, such as diabetes, porphyria, and toxins (e.g., lead). For many patients, no cause can be found for their abdominal pain and psychosocial evaluation may uncover significant stressors or depression.

PATIENT HISTORY

Initial evaluation of the patient presenting with a complaint of abdominal pain includes a detailed description of the pain and its onset, along with assessment of the risks for the different diseases that can cause abdominal pain. Table 1.3 outlines important elements of the history.

Pain Onset

Pain that develops suddenly suggests a vascular cause (e.g., organ infarction, AAA) or perforation or rupture of an abdominal organ. Examples would include perforated ulcer, esophageal rupture, splenic infarction, and dissecting or ruptured AAA. Extraabdominal causes of sudden pain that are referred to the abdomen include myocardial infarction, spontaneous pneumothorax, and ruptured ectopic pregnancy. Onset of pain with peptic ulcer disease, diverticulitis, appendicitis, bowel obstruction, biliary or renal colic, and pancreatitis is generally over minutes to hours. The exact onset of chronic abdominal pain is often difficult to define.

Pain Location

Location of the pain (Table 1.2) can provide the most significant information in directing the workup. Recognition of pain radiation patterns to different regions, such as the midepigastric pain of pancreatitis being referred to the back or the pain of bil-

T ABLE 1.3.   Important elements of the history to evaluate in patients with abdominal pain

Onset of pain
Location of pain
Aggravating/alleviating factors
Associated intestinal symptoms
Associated extraintestinal symptoms
Fever
Past medical and surgical history
Medication use
Family history
Smoking history
Dietary history

iary colic being referred to the scapular region, can assist in determining the cause. Description of the evolution of the pain can also be helpful. For example, the pain of appendicitis can initially be periumbilical, but as the process progresses the pain can be located in the right lower quadrant.

Aggravating or Alleviating Factors

Ingestion of food, passage of bowel movements, or bodily movement can worsen or improve the patient's pain depending on the underlying disease. For example, ingestion of food may alleviate the symptoms of gastroesophageal reflux disease (GERD), but worsen the symptoms associated with bowel obstruction, cholecystitis, pancreatitis, irritable bowel syndrome, and peptic ulcer disease. Passage of bowel movements can bring some relief to patients with bowel obstruction or irritable bowel syndrome. The reclining position can aggravate the symptoms of pancreatitis and GERD. Any body movement can aggravate the pain in conditions with peritoneal inflammation (e.g., appendicitis, diverticulitis, or ruptured viscus). The pain of renal colic occurs independently of the above factors.

Associated Intestinal Symptoms

Nausea and vomiting occur commonly with most conditions causing abdominal pain. Pain that precedes emesis suggests a potential surgical condition, whereas emesis that is followed by pain points more toward a nonsurgical condition. Hematemesis, or "coffee ground" emesis, occurs with peptic ulcer disease, gastritis, esophagitis, or esophageal varices. Diarrhea associated with cramping abdominal pain is present with gastroenteritis, colitis, lactose intolerance, and inflammatory bowel disease. Heme-positive stools can occur with either upper or lower gastrointestinal (GI) blood loss. Heme-positive stools in patients with abdominal pain may be caused by peptic ulcer disease, gastritis, inflammatory bowel disease, infectious colitis, mesenteric ischemia, diverticular disease, or colon cancer. Jaundice in association with abdominal pain suggests liver disease or biliary tract obstruction. Colicky or wavelike discomfort is consistent with an intestinal obstruction. Vomiting is common, particularly in proximal obstruction. More distal obstruction tends to be less painful and associated with less vomiting than proximal obstruction.

Associated Extraintestinal Symptoms

Significant fatigue and weight loss can indicate inflammatory bowel disease or a malignancy as the underlying cause for abdominal pain. Inflammatory bowel disease can have other extraintestinal manifestations such as iritis, arthritis, aphthous ulcers, and dermatologic findings of erythema nodosum and pyoderma gangrenosum. A history of a skin rash that resolved over 7 to 10 days can suggest neuropathic pain of herpes zoster. Referred pain from a cardiac or pulmonary process should be considered if patients complain of shortness of breath, cough, or chest pain. For patients with stigmata of alcohol abuse (e.g., spider hemangioma, palmar erythema, or testicular atrophy), pancreatitis should be considered. In female patients of childbearing age, a missed period may be a clue to ectopic pregnancy. Timing of the pain in relation to the menstrual cycle may point to either endometriosis or mittelschmertz. Finally, vaginal discharge and a history of sexually transmitted disease can indicate the possibility of pelvic inflammatory disease.

Fever

Fever can occur with infectious enteritis, diverticulitis, appendicitis, cholecystitis, intraabdominal abscesses (psoas, subdiaphragmatic), and pulmonary or urinary tract infections. Location of the pain and other associated symptoms can help in further defining the potential sources.

Past Medical and Surgical History

Past medical and surgical history can help in determining possible causes of abdominal pain. For example, patients with known gallstones, nephrolithiasis, or diverticular disease may be experiencing a recurrence. Patients with a history of prior abdominal surgery are at risk for bowel obstruction caused by adhesions. Known hypertension or vascular disease is a risk factor for a vascular cause (e.g., AAA or mesenteric infarction). Causes associated with pancreatitis are presented in Table 1.4. Prior ectopic pregnancies, sexually transmitted disease, or pelvic inflammatory disease may suggest a gynecologic cause. Ketoacidosis can present with abdominal pain and should be considered in diabetics.

Medication Use

Medication use should be reviewed, both for potentially causative agents as well as to assess the patient's attempts at pain relief. Nonsteroidal antiinflammatory medications (NSAIDs) can cause *Helicobacter pylori*-negative ulcer disease. Fenofibrate (Tricor) and gemfibrozil (Lopid) are associated with gallstone formation. Triamterene (Dyrenium) can lead to the formation of renal stones. Azathioprine (Imuran), 6-mercaptopurine (Purinethol), didanosine (Videx), and several other medications can cause pancreatitis (Table 1.5). Many medications can cause GI upset or elevation of hepatic transaminases.

Family History

A family history of inflammatory bowel disease, *H. pylori*-positive peptic ulcer disease, colon cancer, nephrolithiasis, cardiovascular disease, or AAA increases the patient's risk for developing these diseases. Hereditary hypercoagulable states can lead to venous thromboembolic disease and pulmonary embolism with pain referred to the abdomen or, less commonly, to infarction of intraabdominal organs (e.g., mesenteric infarction).

Smoking History

Smoking is associated with the development of peptic ulcer disease and vascular disease, but may be protective for ulcerative colitis.

T ABLE 1.4.   Causes of pancreatitis

Alcohol
Cystic fibrosis
Gallstones
Hereditary
Hypercalcemia
Hypertriglyceridemia
Idiopathic
Infections
    Viruses: mumps, coxsackie B, hepatitis, rubella, Epstein-Barr virus, HIV, cytomegalovirus, varicella
    Bacteria: mycoplasma, campylobacter, leptospira, tuberculosis, legionella
Medications
Pancreas divisum
Penetrating peptic ulcer
Postsurgical or post-ERCP
Trauma

ERCP, endoscopic retrograde cholangiopancreatography; HIV, human immunodeficiency virus.

T ABLE 1.5. Medications reported to cause pancreatitis

6-mercaptopurine (Purinethol)	Methyldopa (Aldomet)	Sulindac (Clinoril)
Azathioprine (Imuran)	Metronidazole (Flagyl)	Tetracycline
Cimetidine (Tagamet)	Pentamidine (Pentam[300])	Thiazide diuretics
Didanosine (Videx)	Ranitidine (Zantac)	Valproic acid (Depacon)
Estrogens	Ritonavir (Norvir)	Zalcitabine (HIVID)
Ethacrynic acid (Endecrin)	Sulfonamides	Zidovudine (Retrovir)
Furosemide (Lasix)		

Dietary History

Ingestion of food can worsen or alleviate abdominal pain, depending on its cause. With GERD and peptic ulcer disease, food may alleviate the pain. With cholecystitis, pancreatitis, mesenteric ischemia, and bowel obstruction, the pain will worsen with ingestion of food. Patients with inflammatory bowel disease exacerbations, diverticulitis, and appendicitis are likely to be anorexic.

PHYSICAL EXAMINATION

Physical examination begins with assessment of the vital signs to determine the stability of the patient. Hypotension can signify AAA, rupture of an intraabdominal organ, significant anemia, dehydration, or sepsis. Fever can occur with appendicitis, diverticulitis, cholecystitis, or urinary tract infection.

A general examination of the patient should be performed, looking for possible disease that can cause pain referred to the abdomen. The patient's appearance and posture can give some useful clues. For example, patients with renal colic or an intestinal obstruction may be restless, whereas patients with peritonitis tend to be still. A patient with pancreatitis may prefer to sit up and lean forward and may be more uncomfortable in the supine position. The chest should be checked for rubs and signs of lower lobe consolidation. The heart should also be examined.

Examination of the abdomen often begins with inspection of the abdomen. Abdominal distention can indicate bowel obstruction. Scars from prior surgeries should be noted. The rash of herpes zoster may be present. Skin discoloration or bruising should be noted, which can indicate retroperitoneal bleeding that can occur with hemorrhagic pancreatitis. Jaundice can indicate biliary disease or hepatitis (Chapter 3).

After inspecting the abdomen, auscultate for bowel sounds. Hyperactive bowel sounds occur with gastroenteritis or partial bowel obstruction, with high-pitched, tinkling bowel sounds being characteristic of the latter. Hypoactive bowel sounds may be present with diverticulitis or appendicitis, and a silent abdomen often indicates generalized peritonitis. Presence of abdominal bruits suggests potential vascular pathology.

Palpation of the abdomen should begin with light palpation in areas away from the abdominal pain. Localization of the pain is helpful in narrowing the differential diagnosis (Table 1.2). For example, a positive Murphy's sign, increased pain on palpation of the right upper quadrant while the patient inspires, is supportive of the diagnosis of cholecystitis. Generalized severe abdominal tenderness indicates diffuse peritoneal inflammation. Significant abdominal pain in the absence of significant physical examination findings is consistent with mesenteric ischemia as a cause. Abdominal guarding, presence of masses, hernias, or organomegaly should be noted during palpation. Test for rebound tenderness by asking the patient to cough.

A rectal examination should be performed to palpate for masses and to check the stool for occult blood. In women, a pelvic examination should be performed to check for pelvic masses, cervical or vaginal discharge, and presence of cervical motion tenderness. In male patients, inspection of the testicles should be part of the physical in the event that pain from testicular torsion or epididymitis is referred to the abdomen.

DIAGNOSTIC STUDIES

Laboratory studies (Table 1.6) should include a complete blood count (CBC), urinalysis, and, in women of childbearing age, a pregnancy test. Additional laboratory tests commonly obtained include liver function tests, amylase, lipase, and basic metabolic panel.

The CBC can indicate the likelihood of a bacterial infection and detect the presence of anemia. It can also confirm the presence of an acute inflammatory process. In elderly patients, the differential is extremely important because a shift to immature forms of white blood cells can indicate significant disease in patients with just mildly elevated or normal white blood counts. The urinalysis may show pyuria or hematuria, thus pointing toward the urinary tract as a potential source of the abdominal pain. Abnormalities in liver function tests and amylase or lipase can signify liver or pancreatic disease. The basic metabolic panel can assess hydration, renal function, and electrolytes. An elevated glucose level may be primary or secondary in relation to a patient's abdominal pain. Elevation of the blood urea nitrogen (BUN) may indicate gastrointestinal bleeding, particularly in the upper GI tract.

Depending on the patient's status and the results of the laboratory studies, radiologic testing may be indicated. Several tests useful in the initial assessment of abdominal pain include the abdominal series of plain radiographs, computed tomography (CT) scan of the abdomen, ultrasound of the abdomen, and intravenous pyelograms.

T ABLE 1.6. Diagnostic testing to evaluate abdominal pain

Test	Purpose
CBC	Identifying anemia or hemorrhage, infection
Urinalysis	Suspected renal infection, renal stones, diabetes
Liver panel	Suspected cholecystitis, hepatitis
Amylase	Suspected pancreatitis
Lipase	Suspected pancreatitis
Serum calcium	Pancreatitis
Basic metabolic panel	Nausea, vomiting, diarrhea; dehydration, impaired renal function, diabetes
Lipids	Pancreatitis
Human chorionic gonadotropin	Women in whom pregnancy/ectopic pregnancy is possible
Plain films	Perforated viscus, bowel obstruction, renal stones
CT scan	Organ infection, infarction or tumor, bowel obstruction, appendicitis, diverticulitis, hemorrhage, AAA, pancreatitis
Ultrasound	Cholecystitis, pancreatitis (initial test), renal infection/obstruction, appendicitis, gynecologic disease, AAA
Intravenous pyelogram	Renal stones, hematuria evaluation

AAA, abdominal aortic aneurysm; CBC, complete blood cell count; CT, computed tomography.

Plain Abdominal Radiographs

Plain films are often obtained; they are useful in evaluating for intestinal obstruction and for free air, which can signify a perforated viscus. The plain film has a sensitivity of 30% to 60% for detecting free air, and is diagnostic for 50% to 60% of cases of bowel obstruction. Additional information from plain films is limited, but can include evidence of either kidney stones or gallstones, fecal impaction, pancreatic calcification caused by chronic pancreatitis, or calcification consistent with an AAA. A chest x-ray study may demonstrate a basilar infiltrate or free air under the diaphragm.

Abdominal Computed Tomography Scans

Computed tomography has become one of the most widely used tests for evaluating undifferentiated acute abdominal pain, as well as pancreatitis, appendicitis, and diverticulitis. The CT scan has a sensitivity and specificity of greater than 90% for both appendicitis and diverticulitis. A CT scan is the most useful radiographic test for visualizing the pancreas in patients with acute disease. Ultrasound can also be used, but is technically inadequate in up to 30% of patients. Integrity of the intraabdominal organs and presence of hemorrhage can be detected after traumatic injury. For patients with diffuse or undifferentiated pain, CT can visualize the intestines, organs, and vessels for evidence of inflammation, obstruction, ischemia, or infarction and help in further directing the evaluation or therapy.

Ultrasound

Ultrasound is commonly used to evaluate patients with abdominal pain and suspected gallstones, renal stones, pyelonephritis, appendicitis, or gynecologic disease. Ultrasound is commonly the first radiologic study performed in patients being evaluated for cholecystitis. Ultrasound can detect the presence of gallstones, gallbladder wall edema, a positive Murphy sign during testing, and the caliber of the biliary ducts. However, hepatobiliary scintigraphy is the most specific test for diagnosing acute cholecystitis. For renal disease, ultrasound can be useful to look for ureteral obstruction; it may show parenchymal evidence of pyelonephritis and abscess formation. With lower quadrant pain, ultrasound is commonly the test first used for women and children because of lower cost and lack of radiation exposure. Ultrasound has a sensitivity of approximately 85% and specificity of approximately 90% for diagnosing appendicitis. Ultrasound is the modality frequently used in assessing the uterus, fallopian tubes, and ovaries for gynecologic disease in patients with abdominal pain.

Intravenous Pyelograms

Intravenous pyelograms are the preferred test for establishing urinary tract obstruction. This test is also of use in evaluating patients with hematuria; after trauma, it can detect renal damage. However, a CT scan will usually be the initial test for patients with abdominal trauma. For patients with renal failure or reactions to contrast media, ultrasound is commonly performed as the initial test to determine presence of obstruction.

RISK FACTORS

Hypertension and known vascular disease are risk factors for vascular causes of abdominal pain (e.g., mesenteric ischemia, organ infarction, and AAA) as well as referred pain from myocardial infarction. In addition, atrial fibrillation is a risk factor for mesenteric artery emboli.

Alcohol use, cigarette smoking, and caffeine use all predispose to the development of GERD. Alcohol use can cause gastritis and pancreatitis. Cigarette smoking has been linked to peptic ulcer disease.

Advancing age is a risk factor for development of vascular disease, cholecystitis, and diverticulitis.

Hyperlipidemia is a risk factor for vascular disease and pancreatitis. Triglyceride values greater than 700 mg/dl place the patient at increased risk for pancreatitis, and often the values in patients with pancreatitis are greater than 1000 mg/dl.

Obesity or a change in weight can predispose to gallstone formation.

Medications have been linked to the development of gastric and duodenal ulcers as well as pancreatitis (Table 1.5).

Hypercalcemia, such as occurs with hyperparathyroidism, can cause pancreatitis.

Abdominal surgery can lead to the formation of adhesions and resultant bowel obstruction. In addition, past history can signify recurrence of disease, such as diverticulitis.

Family history can play a significant role for patients who develop gallstones, kidney stones, colon cancer, inflammatory bowel disease; it may play a role in peptic ulcer disease.

In women, abdominal pain may have a gynecologic cause (e.g., ovarian torsion, endometriosis, ectopic pregnancy, and pelvic inflammatory disease). A history of sexually transmitted disease and prior episodes of pelvic inflammatory disease increase the risk for pelvic inflammatory disease. Women are also at a greater risk of developing cholecystitis.

PATHOPHYSIOLOGY

The pathophysiology of many of these diseases is covered in other chapters within this book. Further discussion in this chapter is limited to pancreatitis, diverticulitis, and appendicitis.

Pancreatitis

Pancreatic proteolytic enzymes are normally secreted from the pancreas in an inactive form into pancreatic ducts and exit the ampulla of Vater to the intestine. Pancreatitis is thought to occur when these enzymes are prematurely activated within the pancreas. The initial inflammatory reaction occurs locally and results in pancreatic inflammation and edema, with the patient's symptoms at this time being primarily midepigastric pain, along with nausea and vomiting. Subsequently, inflammation involves the tissues surrounding the pancreas. For example, retroperitoneal inflammation occurs and the patient experiences pain that radiates through to the back and intensifies in the supine position. Hyperglycemia and hypocalcemia are common metabolic abnormalities occurring with pancreatitis. With more severe forms of pancreatitis, necrosis and hemorrhage can occur, resulting in Cullen's or Grey Turner's sign (bluish periumbilical or flank discoloration). Fluid sequestration within the abdomen and release of chemical mediators into the circulation that affect vascular tone and permeability can lead to shock. Adult respiratory distress syndrome and renal failure can occur. Release of lipase into the circulation can lead to fat necrosis. Other complications of pancreatitis include bacterial pancreatic infection, most commonly caused by enteric organisms, or pseudocyst formation. Pseudocysts form when a pancreatic duct ruptures and pancreatic fluid is secreted into a closed space. Pseudocysts occur in approximately 10% of patients and most resolve spontaneously. Hemorrhage, rupture, or infection of a pseudocyst is associated with increased mortality.

Chronic pancreatitis can occur as a result of recurrent episodes of acute pancreatitis or as a painless process that ultimately results in decreased pancreatic endocrine and exocrine function. In addition to pain, pleural or peritoneal effusions, and pseudocyst formation, patients may develop steatorrhea and diabetes mellitus.

Diverticulitis

The colon consists of four layers of tissue: the mucosa, submucosa, muscle, and serosa. Diverticula are herniations of the mucosa and submucosa through the muscular layer into the serosa. Diverticula occur in association with perforating arteries in the colon, most commonly the sigmoid colon. Diverticulosis is the term applied when a patient has diverticula. This is generally regarded as an asymptomatic condition, although up to 20% of patients may have symptoms consistent with irritable bowel syndrome.

The mucosal layer of the diverticulum can be injured by inspissated food particles or stool, which can lead to the formation of microabscesses. Rupture of these abscesses into the serosa causes inflammation in the immediate area, resulting in diverticulitis. Perforation can also occur into the peritoneal space and cause peritonitis. If diverticulitis occurs contiguous with other structures, then the inflammation can lead to fistula formation (e.g., colovesical fistula). Repetitive episodes of inflammation in the colon and pericolonic tissues can lead to colonic stricture with resultant obstructive symptoms. Bleeding can occur from inflammation and trauma to the penetrating arteries associated with diverticula, but rarely occurs with acute diverticulitis.

Appendicitis

The appendix is a tubular structure located at the posterior aspect of the distal cecum. The opening of the appendix into the cecum can become obstructed by fecaliths, lymphoid tissue hypertrophy, barium, adhesions, stool or food particles, or foreign bodies. When this occurs, mucus continues to be secreted into the lumen of the appendix, and bacterial overgrowth can occur. These two elements combine to increase the pressure within the appendix, which leads to compromise of its vascular supply. Inflammation, bacterial invasion, and ischemia can lead to perforation of the appendix. If this remains contained, then an abscess can result. If perforation occurs into the peritoneal cavity, then generalized peritonitis can result.

DIFFERENTIAL DIAGNOSIS

The differential diagnosis for abdominal pain is presented in Table 1.2 and discussed by clinical presentation in the *Clinical Manifestations* section of this chapter. The following discussion again will be limited to pancreatitis, diverticulitis, and appendicitis because many of the other causes for abdominal pain are discussed in other chapters in this book.

Pancreatitis

Pancreatitis occurs with an incidence of 100 to 200 episodes per million people per year. Most of these patients suffer mild pancreatitis and recover uneventfully. However, 15% to 20% of patients will have severe pancreatitis and may experience complications. It is this group that accounts for the 10% mortality rate associated with pancreatitis. No difference is seen between male or female patients in the incidence of pancreatitis. In 80% of cases of pancreatitis, alcohol or gallstones are the underlying cause. Of patients, 10% have idiopathic pancreatitis. Occult microlithiasis is thought to be the underlying factor in most patients with idiopathic pancreatitis. Rare hereditary autosomal dominant conditions causing pancreatitis have been described. The remainder are attributed to various causes as outlined in Table 1.4.

Onset of midepigastric abdominal pain is the initial symptom in a patient with pancreatitis. This pain is constant and intensifies with radiation to the back. The patient may find it more comfortable to lean forward. Usually, there is associated nausea and vomiting. Fever may also be present, even in the absence of infection. Physical examination will reveal tenderness in the midepigastric region, diminished bowel sounds, and, possibly, abdominal distention.

In more severe pancreatitis a more marked generalized tenderness, signs of shock, such as low blood pressure, rapid heartbeat, tachypnea, and cool extremities may be seen. Jaundice may be present because of obstruction of biliary flow, either from gallstones or pancreatic edema. With hemorrhagic pancreatitis a bluish discoloration of the periumbilical or flank regions as well as abdominal guarding and rebound tenderness may be seen. Painful skin nodules occur rarely.

In 70% to 80% of cases, chronic pancreatitis is related to alcohol abuse. Patients may have persistent or recurrent episodes of epigastric abdominal pain with radiation to the back. Acute worsening of pain may signify an episode of acute pancreatitis superimposed on the chronic disease. As destruction of the gland progresses, the pain may diminish. Steatorrhea and diabetes are consequences of glandular destruction and loss of exocrine and endocrine pancreatic function. The physical examination of the patient with chronic pancreatitis may be normal, other than epigastric tenderness. Pseudocysts, if present, are usually not palpable.

Elevation of the serum amylase and lipase is indicative of pancreatic inflammation. Amylase is more sensitive but less specific than lipase in detecting pancreatitis. Often, however, the two are used together. The amylase is cleared rapidly from the bloodstream (half-life 10 hours) and may return to normal if the patient does not present at the onset of symptoms. Lipase rises slightly later, is cleared slower, and remains elevated longer than amylase. Other causes of elevated amylase are listed in Table 1.7. However, the patient's clinical presentation, evaluation of other studies obtained to evaluate the abdominal pain, use of lipase along with amylase, and, if necessary, measurement of amylase isoenzymes, or amylase to creatinine clearance ratio can determine the cause of an elevated amylase.

During an acute episode of pancreatitis, the white blood cell count (WBC) will often be elevated with presence of a left shift. Hyperglycemia, elevated BUN, hypoalbuminemia, hypertriglyceridemia, hypocalcemia, and abnormal liver enzymes are all common findings. Increased bilirubin and elevated liver enzymes may be caused by

T ABLE 1.7. Causes of serum amylase elevation

Abdominal surgery
Bowel obstruction
Cardiac failure
Common bile duct obstruction (e.g., stones, tumor)
Diabetic ketoacidosis
Intraabdominal hemorrhage
Macroamylasemia
Mesenteric infarction
Pancreatitis
Perforated peptic ulcer
Peritonitis
Post-ERCP or pancreatic trauma
Pregnancy
Renal failure
Salivary gland infection (e.g., mumps)

ERCP, endoscopic retrograde cholangiopancreatography.

T ABLE 1.8.   Criteria for poorer prognosis in patients with pancreatitis

Ranson's criteria	Modified Glascow criteria
Admission	**Within 48 h**
Age > 55 yr	Age > 55 yr
WBC > 16,000/mm^3	WBC > 15,000/mm^3
Glucose > 200 mg/dl	Glucose > 180 mg/dl
LDH > 350 IU/L	BUN > 45 mg/dl
AST > 250 U/L	LDH > 600 IU/L
	Calcium < 8.0 mg/dl
Initial 48 h	Albumin < 3.2 g/dl
HCT decrease by > 10%	Po$_2$ < 60 mm Hg
BUN increase > 5 mg/dl	
Po$_2$ < 60 mm Hg	
Base deficit > 4 mEq/L	
Calcium < 8.0 mg/dl	
Estimated fluid sequestration > 6 L	

AST, aspartate; BUN, blood urea nitrogen; HCT, hematocrit; LDH, lactate dehydrogenase; WBC, white blood cell count; PO$_2$, partial pressure of oxygen.

the pancreatitis or they may indicate that gallstones are the cause of the pancreatitis. Laboratory abnormalities have been studied and developed into scales or criteria (Ranson, Glasgow) to assess prognosis with acute pancreatitis (Table 1.8). As the number of abnormalities or changes increases above two, the mortality rate increases significantly. Laboratory studies for patients with chronic pancreatitis are often normal, with the exception of laboratory signs of malnutrition (decreased lipids, albumin).

Radiographic studies useful in evaluating patients with suspected acute pancreatitis include the plain abdominal radiograph to eliminate bowel obstruction or perforation as considerations. Ultrasound, which is commonly performed initially, is an excellent test to examine the biliary system but is often limited in examination of the pancreas in acute pancreatitis because of overlying bowel. CT of the abdomen is the best radiographic test to detect pancreatitis and can help in determining prognosis. The CT scan is normal in up to 20% of patients with mild disease. Edematous pancreatitis usually follows a favorable course and resolves without complications with supportive care. The mortality rate in these cases is 1% to 3%. Necrotizing pancreatitis (20% of cases) has a higher mortality rate of 10% to 30%, especially if complicated by infection. If infection is suspected, CT-guided aspiration can be performed to assist in guiding therapy. Pseudocysts, if present, can be followed with either ultrasound or CT scan.

Evaluation of chronic pancreatitis may include ultrasound, abdominal CT, endoscopic retrograde cholangiopancreatography (ERCP), or no radiographic testing, depending on the certainty of the diagnosis and its cause.

Diverticulitis

Diverticula occur in up to 10% of patients aged more than 50 years, and may be present in up to 80% of those aged more than 85 years. It has been estimated that up to 20% of patients with diverticula will develop symptomatic disease. More than 80% of the symptomatic patients can be managed as outpatients. Of those requiring hospitalization, 20% or more will require surgical intervention. An approximate 30% chance of recurrence exists after treatment for diverticulitis. With each recurrence of diverticulitis, the patient's risk for subsequent recurrences increases.

The typical presentation of a patient with diverticulitis is with abdominal pain in the left lower quadrant, as 85% of cases involve the sigmoid colon. Associated symptoms can include low-grade fever, nausea, and anorexia. With abscess formation or free perforation, high fever can occur. With free perforation, signs of generalized peritonitis will be present.

An elevated WBC would be the only typical laboratory finding, with more significant elevation with abscess formation or peritonitis. Plain abdominal x-ray study can help exclude other diagnoses. The abdominal CT scan is the most useful radiographic test in identifying diverticulitis as well as the complications (e.g., fistula or abscess formation).

Appendicitis

Appendicitis occurs in 7% of patients during their lifetime. The peak incidence of disease is in persons aged less than 20 years; 80% of patients are aged less than 50 years. However, the rupture and mortality rates are highest in geriatric patients. Patients aged more than 60 years account for 50% of the deaths from appendicitis.

Patients presenting with appendicitis initially have periumbilical abdominal pain that then localizes to the right lower quadrant. The patient may lie motionless with the right thigh flexed. Accompanying symptoms include anorexia, nausea, and vomiting. With appendicitis, abdominal pain typically precedes the vomiting. A low-grade fever may also be present. If perforation or abscess formation occurs, then high fever may be present. Peritoneal signs indicate free perforation. Physical examination is remarkable for tenderness in the right lower quadrant (McBurney's point) along with guarding. Rebound tenderness may also be present.

An elevated WBC is the typical laboratory finding with appendicitis. Plain abdominal radiographs again may be useful in eliminating bowel obstruction or perforation as diagnostic possibilities. An abdominal CT scan is the most reliable radiographic test in detecting appendicitis, which can also detect the presence of an abscess. Ultrasound is also commonly used, particularly in women and children.

REFERRAL

Although mild pancreatitis can be managed on an outpatient basis, most patients are hospitalized for hydration and monitoring until symptoms resolve. For patients with severe or complicated pancreatitis and those with gallstones as the underlying cause, surgical or gastroenterology consultation is warranted. With a pseudocyst or peripancreatic fluid, and concerns regarding bacterial infection, CT-guided aspiration and culture may be needed to direct therapy. Chronic pancreatitis is managed on an outpatient basis, with testing and GI consultation dictated by the certainty of the diagnosis and underlying cause. Exacerbations of chronic pancreatitis will often require hospitalization, as does acute pancreatitis.

Diverticulitis is most often treated on an outpatient basis, and laboratory and radiographic studies can be obtained on an ambulatory basis. Those patients for whom the diagnosis is uncertain may benefit from specialist GI or surgical consultation on an outpatient basis. After symptoms resolve, referral for colonoscopy is suggested to ensure that an underlying neoplasm is not responsible for the patient's symptoms.

Patients with more severe symptoms of diverticulitis are hospitalized and surgical consultation is often requested. The rate of surgical intervention is higher in this group. Indications for surgical intervention can include presence of peritonitis, fistula, persistent bowel obstruction, or abscesses. For patients with abscesses, interventional radiology consultation can be obtained for CT-guided drainage of an abscess.

Appendicitis is a surgical condition and requires hospital admission and surgical consultation for timely evaluation and surgical treatment. Again, if an abscess has formed, initial therapy may involve CT-guided drainage and antibiotics.

MANAGEMENT

Pancreatitis

Patients with acute pancreatitis (Table 1.9) are typically hospitalized, take nothing by mouth to limit stimulation of pancreatic enzyme secretion, and are provided with intravenous hydration and pain medication until symptoms resolve. Monitoring for onset of shock, infection; and respiratory, renal, and fluid or electrolyte

T ABLE 1.9. Treatment of acute pancreatitis

SUPPORTIVE MEASURES
Intravenous hydration
Nothing by mouth until pain subsides, pancreatic enzymes decline
Pain medication (e.g., meperidine)
Monitor for complications

COMPLICATIONS
Local

Necrosis	
Sterile	Supportive measures and possibly surgical debridement; prophylactic antibiotics of unproven value
Infected	Surgical debridement, antibiotics
Abscess	Surgical drainage, antibiotics
Pseudocyst	Monitor for persistence or size, >6 wk/6 cm. Drainage may be indicated to prevent complications

Systemic

Hypocalcemia	Check ionized calcium or albumin; replace if true hypocalcemia or clinical signs (e.g., Chvostek's sign, tetany)
Hyperglycemia	Insulin
Hypotension	Aggressive hydration (up to 6–10 L in 24 h)
Renal failure	Fluid restriction, pressor agents if low blood pressure; possibly hemodialysis
Shock	Aggressive hydration, pressor agents, central venous or Swan-Ganz monitoring in intensive care unit
Respiratory failure or acute respiratory distress syndrome	Oxygen, ventilatory support
Disseminated intravascular coagulation	Provide blood products (red blood cells, fresh frozen plasma, cryoprecipitate, platelets) as dictated by laboratory or clinical state

POSSIBLE INDICATIONS FOR SURGERY
Gallstones
Necrosis with infection or suspected infection
Necrosis without clinical improvement or with clinical decline
Abscess
Persistent or enlarging pseudocyst
Increasing fluid collection in symptomatic patient
Massive bleeding

abnormalities with timely treatment are the cornerstone of therapy. Aggressive intravenous hydration is warranted, particularly for severe pancreatitis, to replace intravascular volume lost because of fluid shifts. Nasogastric tubes are useful only in instances of vomiting or persistent ileus. If infection is suspected, then CT-guided aspiration and culture of necrotic tissue may be indicated along with antibiotic therapy. Pain management often involves the use of narcotic medications. Meperidine (Demerol) is often used. Morphine should not be routinely used as it can cause spasm at Oddi's sphincter. As the patient clinically improves and the pancreatic enzymes return to normal, food can be introduced. Typically, this is a clear liquid diet, which is advanced as tolerated. Currently, no consensus exists on whether a special diet (i.e., high-carbohydrate, low-fat, low-protein) has any impact on patient outcome.

Patients with chronic pancreatitis can have chronic pain, steatorrhea, and diabetes as problems that may require therapy. Chronic pain should initially be treated with non-narcotic pain medication. If the pain persists, then narcotic medications are recommended, along with monitoring the patient's use of these medications for potential abuse. Even in the absence of clinical signs of malabsorption, pancreatic enzyme therapy can be provided to attempt to alleviate pain. Refractory pain may require nerve blocks or surgical interventions.

Steatorrhea is managed by the use of pancreatic enzymes with each meal. Pancreatic enzymes, in particular lipase, are degraded and deactivated by gastric acid. Enteric and nonenteric preparations have been developed. The difference between the two is that the enteric-coated preparations release their enzymes at a pH of 5.5, thus, theoretically, delaying their release and resisting gastric deactivation. Typically, a patient is started on a nonenteric-coated preparation (e.g., Viokase); if with dosage titration, symptoms persist, then an enteric-coated preparation may be tried. In some patients the pH may rise with ingestion of food, and then drop and allow degradation of either preparation. In this instance, acid suppression (use of a a histamine$_2$ [H$_2$] blocker or proton pump inhibitor) along with a nonenteric-coated preparation may be helpful. If symptoms still persist, then consultation and consideration of other causes (e.g., bacterial overgrowth) should ensue. Insulin and dietary measures are used to manage patients with diabetes.

Patients with acute or chronic pancreatitis can develop pseudocysts as a complication of their disease. Although pseudocysts can resolve spontaneously, those present for more than 6 weeks are less likely to resolve spontaneously. Pseudocysts that are more than 5 cm in size have an increased rate of complications that include rupture, hemorrhage, or infection. Ultrasound or CT can be used to monitor the presence and size of pseudocysts. For patients at increased risk of complications, surgical or gastroenterology consultation should be considered for possible operative or endoscopic surgical drainage.

Diverticulitis

Patients with mild diverticulitis are managed as outpatients with antibiotics, directed at gram-negative rods and anaerobes (Table 1.10). Additionally, patients can be placed on a clear liquid diet, with advancement of the diet as tolerated if clinical improvement is noted within the following 2 to 3 days. Antibiotic therapy is continued for 7 to 14 days. Outpatient evaluation (CT scan) and follow-up colonoscopy are often recommended. To prevent further episodes, fiber supplements or a higher-fiber diet are prescribed.

Patients requiring hospitalization are given nothing by mouth, and provided with intravenous hydration and antibiotics. Surgical consultation and CT scan are obtained, and the patient is monitored for complications. As the pain and symptoms resolve, a clear liquid diet is provided and advanced as tolerated. The patient is then discharged

T ABLE 1.10. Examples of antibiotic coverage for diverticulitis and appendicitis

Outpatient/Oral (for diverticulitis)	• Trimethoprim/sulfamethoxazole 160/800 mg bid OR ciprofloxacin (Cipro), 500 mg bid PLUS metronidazole (Flagyl), 500 mg qid • Amoxicillin/clavulanic acid (Augmentin), 500 mg tid or 875 mg bid
Inpatient/Intravenous	• Ciprofloxacin (Cipro), 400 mg IV q12h OR gentamicin (Garamycin),2.0 mg/kg loading dose then 1.7 mg/kg IV q8h OR cefotaxime (Claforan), 2.0 g IV q4–8h OR aztreonam (Azactam), 2.0 g IV q8h PLUS metronidazole (Flagyl), 500 mg IV q6h OR clindamycin 450–900 mg IV q8h • Ampicillin/sulbactam (Unasyn), 3.0 g IV q6h • Cefoxitin (Mefoxin), 2.0 g IV q8h • Cefotetan (Cefotan), 2.0 g IV q12h • Ticarcillin/clavulanic acid (Timentin), 3.1 g IV q6h • Piperacillin/tazobactam (Zosyn), 3.375 g IV q6h

bid, two times per day; IV, intravenous; q, every day; qid, four times per day; tid, three times a day.

on oral antibiotics, again for a course of 7 to 14 days. Preventive and follow-up testing are as noted above.

Appendicitis

Appendicitis is a surgical condition, and surgical consultation should be obtained before proceeding with therapy. In the interim, the patient should be given nothing by mouth and provided with intravenous hydration and antibiotics (Table 1.10). Approximately 20% of surgically removed appendices are normal, and the patient's abdominal pain is subsequently attributed to another cause. This rate is considered acceptable in order to prevent the complications resulting from delay of surgery for true appendicitis.

Patients who develop abscesses can initially be treated with CT-guided drainage and antibiotics. After symptoms improve, the patient can be discharged from the hospital on antibiotic therapy, with readmission at a later date (commonly, 6 weeks) for appendectomy.

FOLLOW-UP

Patients with pancreatitis should be advised to report further episodes of pain and onset of fever. Abnormal laboratory test results that can indicate pancreatitis should be repeated after resolution of the acute attack. If an underlying treatable cause is found for the patient's acute pancreatitis (e.g., hyperlipidemia, hypercalcemia), then further evaluation and treatment of that condition should be undertaken. In patients with idiopathic pancreatitis, ERCP may be indicated to complete the evaluation.

Patients with chronic pancreatitis should be monitored for pain control, steatorrhea, and diabetes. If a pseudocyst is present, then monitoring for symptoms and increasing size or persistence of the cyst is warranted. Ultrasound or CT scan are the radiologic tests used to monitor pseudocysts. Endoscopic or surgical drainage or removal may be indicated if the pseudocyst has been present for more than 6 weeks or is greater than 5 cm in size. In cases where the cause of the patient's chronic pancreatitis is in question, then ERCP may be indicated. ERCP may also be performed if the patient experiences persistent pain or if surgical intervention is being considered. Stent placement is sometimes used to alleviate pain with chronic pancreatitis.

Initial follow-up of patients with diverticulitis being treated as outpatients should be done within 48 to 72 hours to document clinical improvement. Hospitalized patients should be tolerating a diet and be stable on oral medications before discharge. Patients with diverticulitis should undergo a follow-up colonoscopy to ensure that the symptoms are not cancer related.

Follow-up of the patient with appendicitis involves documenting wound healing, and suture or staple removal. No additional follow-up care or evaluation is necessary in the absence of complications.

PATIENT EDUCATION

Patients with pancreatitis should be counseled regarding the potential causes of pancreatitis. If alcohol is a trigger or potential causative factor, then provide information regarding abstinence and resources for substance abuse counseling and support. Patients with acute or chronic pancreatitis should be counseled to report any additional or new abdominal pain as well as fevers. Patients with chronic pancreatitis who are diabetic will need education regarding their diabetes, including information about a low-fat, diabetic diet, glucose monitoring, and insulin or oral hypoglycemic therapy.

Recurrent symptoms of abdominal pain or fever should be reported by patients with diverticulitis or appendicitis, as they may signify abscess formation or recurrent diverticular disease. Instructions to increase dietary fiber may be helpful for patients with diverticular disease.

SUGGESTED READING

Ferzoco LB, Raptopoulos V, Silen W. Acute diverticulitis. *N Engl J Med* 1998;338: 1521–1526.

Grendell JH, Cello JP. Chronic pancreatitis. In: Sleisenger MH, Fordtran JS, eds. *Gastrointestinal disease: pathophysiology, diagnosis, management*, 5th ed. Philadelphia: WB Saunders; 1993:1654–1677.

Gupta PK, al-Kawas FH. Acute pancreatitis: diagnosis and management. *Am Fam Physician* 1995;52:534–543.

Martiin RF, Rossi RL. The acute abdomen: an overview and algorithms. *Surg Clin North Am* 1997;77:1227–1243.

Schrock TR. Acute appendicitis. In: Sleisenger MH, Fordtran JS, eds. *Gastrointestinal disease: pathophysiology, diagnosis, management*, 5th ed. Philadelphia: WB Saunders; 1993:1339–1345.

Recurrent Abdominal Pain in Children

Sanford R. Kimmel and William B. Klein

DEFINITION

Recurrent abdominal pain (RAP) occurs in 10% to 15% of children aged between 4 and 16 years. It is defined as episodic pain that occurs for longer than 3 months and affects normal activity. The pain is real but may be isolated and paroxysmal, accompanied by dyspepsia, or associated with an altered bowel pattern. It is often caused by a functional bowel disorder. The child may refuse to go to school or be sent home from school because of persisting pain. Children aged less than 4 years who have chronic abdominal pain require a more detailed evaluation to exclude organic causes.

CLINICAL MANIFESTATIONS

Boyle has characterized RAP into three patterns as listed below.

Isolated Paroxysmal Pain

Isolated paroxysmal pain is typically vague in character, variable in severity, and periumbilical in location. It lasts less than 1 hour in 50% of children and less than 3 hours in another 40%. Less than 10% of children have continuous pain. The pain seldom radiates and is unrelated to meals or activity. It often occurs in the evening and interferes with the child's ability to fall asleep, but rarely wakes up the sleeping child. During a painful attack, the child may double over and cry. More than 50% of children have associated symptoms such as headache, nausea, dizziness, and fatigue.

Abdominal Pain Associated with Dyspepsia

Abdominal pain associated with dyspepsia is located in the epigastrium, and right or left upper quadrant. It can be accompanied by episodic vomiting. Symptoms are usually related to meals and can include anorexia, nausea, early satiety, postprandial abdominal bloating, indigestion, and belching.

Abdominal Pain with Altered Bowel Pattern

Abdominal pain with altered bowel pattern is typically variable in severity and localized to the lower abdomen. Diarrhea, constipation, or a sense of incomplete evacuation follows a bowel movement, which can relieve or worsen the pain. Functional irritable bowel syndrome (IBS) is the most common cause of this pattern.

PATIENT HISTORY

Apley reports that an organic cause was found in less than 10% of children with RAP. He also notes: "The further the localization of the pain from the umbilicus, the more likely is there to be an underlying organic disorder." Children should be asked about the location of their pain by having them point at it with one finger. However, many younger children with RAP will not be able to localize the pain. Older children may be able to characterize the pain as burning, sharp, dull, or cramping. Younger children can be asked if it feels like their stomach is "on fire," if it feels like they have been "stuck with a needle," or if the pain causes them to double over. Elicit information about the timing of the pain (e.g., its relationship to meals or waking up at night). Also inquire about factors that make the pain better or worse.

Pain Location

Vague, periumbilical pain is usually functional but can result from other causes, especially fecal impaction. Pain localized to the epigastrium, or right or left upper quadrants, is characteristic of dyspepsia or peptic ulcer disease, especially if accompanied by episodic vomiting. Continuous, midepigastric, or periumbilical pain that radiates to the back suggests pancreatitis. Children with RAP rarely describe radiation of the pain. Recurrent biliary colic caused by cholecystitis or cholelithiasis localizes to the right upper quadrant or epigastrium and frequently follows a meal. Lower abdominal pain, accompanied by diarrhea alternating with constipation, or a sense of incomplete evacuation of the colon is commonly caused by IBS.

Timing of the Pain

Functional abdominal pain usually begins gradually and lasts less than 3 hours. It often occurs in the evening and may prevent the child from falling asleep; however, it rarely awakens the child. Nocturnal pain is suggestive of acid-peptic disease. Gastroesophageal reflux disease (GERD) is suggested by heartburn or indigestion that worsens with lying down or ingesting acidic foods or drinks. It is helpful to ask caregivers or older children to keep a diary listing the child's diet and symptoms, and when the symptoms occur.

Associated Gastrointestinal Symptoms

Irritable bowel syndrome is associated with passing mucus and a feeling of bloating or abdominal distention. Diarrhea, bloating, and increased flatulence likewise can occur with lactose intolerance. Abdominal pain accompanied by diarrhea is the most frequent symptom of Crohn's disease, whereas abdominal pain accompanied by rectal bleeding is most common in ulcerative colitis. However, gastrointestinal (GI) bleeding occurs in some patients with Crohn's disease.

Review of Systems

Fever, anorexia, and weight loss indicate an organic disorder, whereas normal appetite and weight gain suggest a functional cause of RAP. Decreased linear growth and peripheral arthritis of the large joints can occur in both Crohn's disease and ulcerative colitis. Symptoms of dyspepsia include nausea, vomiting, early satiety, and excessive hiccups or belching. GERD can cause chronic cough, laryngitis, or reactive airway disease. Table 2.1 lists "red flags" that strongly suggest an organic cause of RAP.

Family History

A family history of peptic ulcer disease, IBS, inflammatory bowel disease, gallbladder disease, lactose intolerance, other GI disorders, or migraine can provide clues to the diagnosis.

Psychosocial History

The child and the caregivers should be asked if the pain interferes with normal activities. If so, does the child experience secondary gain such as missing school or

T ABLE 2.1.   Red flags in the history that suggest an organic cause of abdominal pain

- Age <4 yrs
- Fever ≥38°C (100.4°F)
- Persistent vomiting
- Pain awakens child at night
- Presence of blood in emesis or stool
- Pain localized away from the umbilicus
- Loss of weight or decreased growth velocity
- Symptoms such as rash, joint pain, dysuria
- Positive family history of inflammatory bowel disease or peptic ulcer disease

Adapted from Boyle JT. Recurrent abdominal pain: an update. *Pediatr Rev* 1997;18:314; with permission.

increased attention? Are there family stresses (e.g., marital difficulties leading to the possibility of divorce or separation)? Sexual abuse should always be considered, and a confidential sexual history should be elicited from older children and adolescents.

PHYSICAL EXAMINATION

Growth Parameters

Recurrent abdominal pain that is accompanied by anorexia, weight loss, or a decrease in linear growth is highly indicative of an underlying organic disorder such as inflammatory bowel disease or malignancy. Normal appetite and growth are suggestive of a functional cause.

General Observation

If the child is complaining of pain at the time of examination, note whether he or she appears to be uncomfortable. If the child can walk, run, or climb on the examining table without apparent discomfort, then a significant organic problem is less likely. On the other hand, a child who moves slowly in a guarded fashion or is doubled over clearly needs a thorough evaluation to exclude organic causes.

Abdominal Examination

A general physical examination should be performed with particular emphasis on the abdomen. Ascultate the abdomen for the presence and activity of bowel sounds. Gently palpate the abdomen for the presence of organomegaly or masses. Areas of tenderness on light or deep palpation should be localized and the presence of rebound or rigidity noted. Care must be taken to avoid undue discomfort to the child that will interfere with further examination. A rectal examination is usually necessary and stool is obtained for occult blood. The presence of GI bleeding suggests a variety of causes including *Helicobacter pylori* gastritis, peptic ulcer disease, or inflammatory bowel disease.

Gynecologic Examination

A pelvic examination should be strongly considered in adolescent girls to check for intrauterine or ectopic pregnancy, sexually transmitted diseases, ovarian masses, or other gynecologic disorders.

DIAGNOSTIC STUDIES

Most children presenting with a history of recurrent abdominal pain should have the following studies: a complete blood count (CBC), erythrocyte sedimentation rate (ESR), urinalysis, and stool for ova and parasites. A urine culture should also be done for children who have urinary symptoms (e.g., dysuria or frequency). Because preschool children and developmentally delayed children may not complain of these symptoms, it is prudent to obtain a urine culture in them as well. Further diagnostic studies are suggested by the pattern of pain and associated symptoms. However, care must be taken to avoid excessive testing because this can increase parental anxiety in addition to putting the child through unnecessary studies.

Blood Tests

Blood tests beyond a CBC and ESR must be ordered judiciously, depending on the presenting symptoms. The presence of upper quadrant pain may indicate the need for serum amylase, lipase, and transaminase levels to help rule out pancreatic or hepatic diseases. The decision to obtain an assay for *H. pylori* is controversial. Although *H. pylori* has been found in children with antral nodular gastritis, it is also present in many asymptomatic children and is weakly or inconsistently associated with RAP in children.

Radiographic Studies

When paroxysmal periumbilical pain is accompanied by historical "red flags" (Table 2.1), anemia, an elevated ESR, or blood in the stool, an upper GI series with small bowel follow-through is useful to detect problems such as partial small bowel obstruction, malrotation, or lymphoma. Ultrasonography is rarely useful except when an underlying cholelithiasis or renal abnormality is suspected. Pelvic ultrasound is helpful to evaluate suspected gynecologic problems such as cystic teratoma of the ovary, ectopic pregnancy, and pelvic inflammatory disease.

Endoscopy

Upper endoscopy is most likely to be of benefit in those children presenting with abdominal pain accompanied by dyspepsia. It is the most sensitive test for evaluating inflammatory disease resulting in ulceration, stricture, antral nodular gastritis, and the gastric rugal hypertrophy of Ménétrier's disease (hypertrophic gastritis). In adolescents, it may be reasonable to postpone upper endoscopy for 4 to 6 weeks pending completion of a therapeutic trial of antacids or histamine$_2$ receptor antagonists (H$_2$-blockers). Children aged younger than 12 years presenting with symptoms of dyspepsia should undergo endoscopy. Colonoscopy should be performed in children with unexplained GI bleeding, or signs and symptoms or a family history of inflammatory bowel disease.

Stool Studies

Although usually self-limited, *Giardia lamblia* infection can recur or become chronic. Stool for ova and parasites should be obtained when crampy abdominal pain is accompanied by diarrhea, weight loss, steatorrhea, or lactose intolerance. Children with abdominal pain accompanied by watery diarrhea who were recently exposed to antibiotics should have an assay for *Clostridium difficile* toxin.

Tests for Food Intolerance

Dietary restriction using a lactose-free diet for 2 weeks followed by a lactose challenge is the most convenient method of diagnosing lactose intolerance. If results are equivocal, the lactose breath hydrogen test is more sensitive than the oral tolerance test. Restriction of fructose-containing beverages (e.g., juice or soda pop) or sorbitol-containing products (e.g., sugar-free gum) may also be considered as part of a therapeutic trial.

RISK FACTORS

Boys and girls with RAP are equally affected up to age 9 years. Between ages 9 and 12 years, girls are 1.5 times more likely to have RAP. Otherwise, children with organic pain and functional pain cannot be distinguished on the basis of personality or intelligence. Lactase deficiency is most common in Asian, African-American, and Hispanic children. Crohn's disease and ulcerative colitis are more common in whites, especially those of Jewish descent. *G. lamblia* infection occurs in travelers who drink contaminated water from mountain streams, but can also occur in institutional settings such as day-care centers. *C. difficile* enterocolitis has occurred as a result of exposure to almost all antibiotics.

PATHOPHYSIOLOGY

The causes of functional abdominal pain producing RAP are not well understood. Visceral hypersensitivity, especially to mechanical stimuli can play a role. Visceral afferent nerve fibers enter the dorsal horn of the spinal cord with afferent fibers from corresponding dermatomal segments. Stimulation of visceral afferents may then produce referred pain while other impulses are transmitted to the cerebral cortex. According to the gate theory of pain, larger-diameter afferent fibers can modulate these signals such that pain is not perceived. However, circumstances such as anxiety or stressful life events can inhibit modulation such that even normal intestinal sensation is perceived as pain.

Altered gut motility can be manifested as increased intensity of intestinal muscle contraction in both the small and large bowels, accompanied by prolonged intestinal transit times. However, findings are inconsistent, and increased parasympathetic tone and gut motility have also been demonstrated. Associated symptoms such as headache, pallor, and dizziness suggest a dysfunction of the autonomic nervous system in some patients.

It has also been suggested that RAP may have some psychological causes. Previous allegations that children with RAP are compulsive, high strung, or perfectionists have not been proved in controlled studies. Children with RAP demonstrate increased anxiety, but no more than children with organic diseases. Family members often have a high frequency of painful complaints such as IBS, peptic ulcer, or migraine headaches. Some children with RAP associated with vomiting and a family history of migraine are diagnosed as having "abdominal migraines" that may respond to migraine treatments.

DIFFERENTIAL DIAGNOSIS

The differential diagnosis of RAP is extensive. Table 2.2 summarizes some of the more significant or common considerations in evaluating children with this problem.

REFERRAL

Referral for further evaluation and workup may be required in cases of diagnostic uncertainty. Children with dyspepsia may benefit from referral for upper endoscopy, especially if they do not respond to an empiric trial of treatment with H_2-blockers. Children who present with "red flags" such as passage of blood in emesis or stool and

T ABLE 2.2. Significant causes of recurrent abdominal pain

Disorder	History	Physical
Gastrointestinal		
Peptic ulcer disease	Epigastric burning, history of NSAID use	Epigastric tenderness
Gastroesophageal reflux disease	Heartburn aggravated by lying down or acidic foods, odynophagia	Epigastric tenderness
Chronic pancreatitis	Epigastric or back pain, weight loss, steatorrhea	Epigastric tenderness
Cholelithiasis	RUQ pain, worse with meals	RUQ tenderness, positive Murphy's sign
Choledochal cyst	RUQ pain, vomiting	RUQ mass, jaundice
Lactose intolerance	Bloating, gaseousness, colicky abdominal pain, diarrhea	Abdominal distention
Crohn's disease	Fever, weight loss, diarrhea, abdominal pain, rectal bleeding, family history	Abdominal tenderness, perianal skin tags, fistula or abscess, growth failure
Ulcerative colitis	Rectal bleeding, abdominal pain, diarrhea, family history	Abdominal distention and tenderness, uveitis, mouth sores
Malrotation and volvulus	Bilious vomiting	Distended tender abdomen, rectal bleeding
Inguinal hernia	Swelling in inguinal area, labia or scrotum, emesis	Palpable hernia, abdominal distention
Constipation	Colicky abdominal pain, associated enuresis	Palpable stool LLQ, impacted stool on rectal examination
Intermittent intussusception	Colicky pain, emesis, blood and mucus in stool, currant-jelly stool	Mass on abdominal or rectal examination often in RUQ, abdominal distention
Meckel's diverticulum	Painless rectal bleeding, RLQ pain only with obstruction or peptic ulceration	Occasionally RLQ tenderness
Appendiceal colic	Episodic RLQ tenderness	RLQ tenderness without peritoneal signs
Henoch-Schönlein purpura	Rash, colicky abdominal pain, arthritis, GI bleeding	Palpable purpura, abdominal tenderness, hematuria
Postsurgical adhesions	Abdominal pain, bilious vomiting	Abdominal distention, hyperactive bowel sounds
Hereditary angioedema	Crampy pain, swelling of face or airway, episodes last 1–4 days	Swelling face, pharynx, genitalia
Infectious		
Parasites (esp. *Giardia*)	Watery diarrhea, cramping, abdominal pain, nausea, anorexia, bloating	Weight loss, decreased growth, abdominal distention

continued

T ABLE 2.2 *continued.* Significant causes of recurrent abdominal pain

Disorder	History	Physical
Helicobacter pylori gastritis	Epigastric pain, postprandial vomiting, anorexia, weight loss	Epigastric tenderness
Bacterial enterocolitis, (*Yersinia, Campylobacter, Clostridium difficile*)	Fever, nausea, abdominal pain, diarrhea, bloody stool, antibiotic exposure	Diffuse or RLQ abdominal pain (esp. *Yersinia*)
Urogenital		
Ureteropelvic junction obstruction	Periumbilical or midepigastric crampy pain with episodic vomiting	Palpable renal mass, UTI hematuria
Primary dysmenorrhea	Cramping, dull, midline, lower abdominal pain with onset of menses, nausea, low back pain	Unremarkable pelvic examination
Endometriosis	Chronic pelvic pain	Nodularity in cul-de-sac
Cystic teratoma	Prepubertal RLQ or LLQ pain	RLQ or LLQ abdominal mass
Ectopic pregnancy	Delayed menses, vaginal bleeding, severe RLQ or LLQ abdominal pain	Adnexal mass
Pelvic inflammatory disease	Lower abdominal pain, vaginal discharge	Cervical motion tenderness, adnexal tenderness
Hematology/Oncology		
Lymphoma	Fever, night sweats, weight loss, pruritus	Lymphadenopathy, hepatomegaly, splenomegaly
Sickle cell vaso-occlusive crisis	Severe abdominal pain	Joint and bone pain or swelling
Neurology		
Abdominal migraines	Paroxysmal abdominal pain, family history of migraines, cyclic vomiting, with or without headache	
Endocrine/Metabolic/Toxic		
Diabetic ketoacidosis	Nausea, vomiting, lethargy, polyuria, polydipsia	Dry mucous membranes, fruity odor, abdominal tenderness
Acute intermittent porphyria	Severe abdominal pain, vomiting, psychiatric disturbances	Abdominal distention, ileus, port wine urine
Lead poisoning (lead colic)	Sporadic vomiting, intermittent abdominal pain, constipation	Developmental delay, with or without anemia

GI, gastrointestinal; LLQ, left lower quadrant; NSAID, nonsteroidal antiinflammatory drug; RUQ, right upper quadrant; RLQ, right lower quadrant; UTI, urinary tract infection.

decrease in weight or growth velocity often require colonoscopy to rule out inflammatory bowel disease. If the physician is reasonably confident that the abdominal pain is functional, then psychological referral to teach the child how to cope with stress and the parents how to manage pain behaviors may be helpful.

MANAGEMENT

An organic cause will not be identified for most children presenting with RAP. However, spontaneous remission occurs in up to 40% of children. It is important to explain to parents (and older children) what is known—not just provide simple reassurance that all is well. Apley stresses that "there should be no reassurance without explanation." In some patients, symptoms can persist into adulthood. Dietary fiber therapy may alleviate the constipation found in more than 20% of children with RAP but may not relieve the abdominal pain. Limiting the intake of milk products, carbonated beverages, or sorbitol-containing products may be helpful in decreasing pain, bloating, and diarrhea. Many children who are lactose-intolerant will respond to a lactose-free diet, but not all children with RAP do so. Because children with both functional and organic causes of RAP experience higher levels of anxiety than normal, stress management training may be helpful because it enables the child and parents to develop skills for coping with stress and pain.

Isolated Paroxysmal Pain

Educate parents and those involved in the child's daily activities that the child's pain is real but that it is important to continue normal activities such as school attendance, even if pain is present. Where possible, environmental stresses that can provoke pain should be identified and minimized. The child should learn how to manage stress and cope with pain. Fiber can be tried, but excessive fiber can increase gas and abdominal distention. If lactose deficiency is confirmed by dietary elimination or a lactose breath hydrogen test, dairy products can be pretreated with lactase enzyme. Fructose or sorbitol can also be eliminated from the diet if these are believed to be culprits in promoting the abdominal pain. Antispasmodics are thought to reinforce the pain behavior but can be useful for occasional short-term use.

Recurrent Abdominal Pain Associated with Dyspepsia

Education and environmental and dietary modifications are recommended for children with functional dyspepsia. Caffeine, fatty foods, and nonsteroidal antiinflammatory drugs should be avoided. Older children with ulcerlike dyspepsia may be treated with an H_2-blocker for 4 to 6 weeks. If not previously performed, upper endoscopy should be done in those children who do not respond to therapy. Prokinetic agents, such as metoclopromide (Reglan), sometimes have been used but are not approved by the US Food and Drug Administration for use in children. More importantly, metoclopromide can, in rare cases, cause dystonic reactions.

Recurrent Abdominal Pain with Altered Bowel Pattern

The treatment approach for isolated paroxysmal pain can be used. However, an antimotility agent such as loperamide (Imodium-AD) can be tried if diarrhea is the predominant symptom. Bulk laxatives, stool softeners, or lactulose may be considered if constipation is the prevailing symptom. Excessive gas can be managed by decreasing intake of carbonated beverages, beans, cabbage, and fructose-sweetened drinks. Simethicone (Mylicon) may relieve gas in some patients. Figure 2.1 summarizes the evaluation and management of the child with RAP.

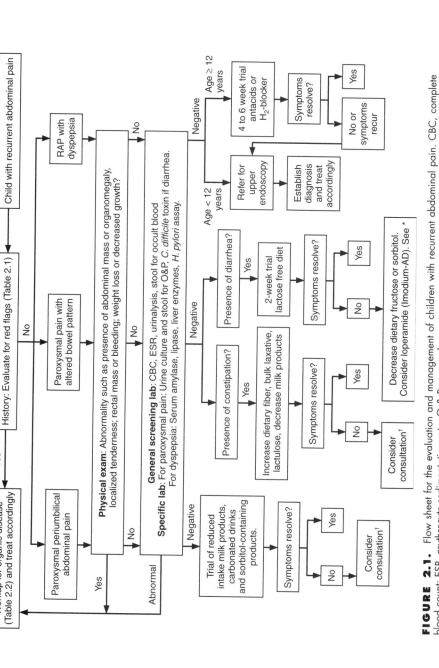

FIGURE 2.1. Flow sheet for the evaluation and management of children with recurrent abdominal pain. CBC, complete blood count; ESR, erythrocyte sedimentation rate; O & P, ova and parasites.

*Children with functional recurrent abdominal pain and their parents should be encouraged to continue normal activity, (including school attendance), decrease environmental stresses, and learn methods to reduce stress and cope with pain.

†Consultation may be helpful in children whose pain persists for more than 3 to 6 weeks, whose symptoms are troublesome, and in those who do not respond to diet manipulation, fever, or therapeutic trial.

FOLLOW-UP

Children with functional RAP require periodic follow-up to ensure that they remain active in school and at home. They and their families must learn to cope with the pain by finding methods to alleviate stress and avoid any secondary gain that comes from focusing on the abdominal pain and associated symptoms. Although organic disease is seldom masked, be alert to any change in symptoms that warrants reevaluation. Fortunately, functional abdominal pain resolves in 30% to 50% of children within 6 weeks of diagnosis.

Potential Problems and Complications

Many children with RAP continue to experience abdominal pain for several years after the initial evaluation. They have higher levels of functional disability, including school absences and use of health services. Higher levels of life stress, especially in girls, are associated with an increased risk of developing IBS during adolescence and young adulthood.

PATIENT EDUCATION

It is important to reassure the child and parents that major life-threatening illnesses have been excluded by the examination. However, it must be emphasized that the pain that the child is experiencing is real and not "just in his/her head." Explain that the reason for the pain is not completely understood, but may be caused by the child being more sensitive to normal GI sensations or to increased GI activity. The child should be encouraged to resume normal activities. Parents can comfort and reassure the child, but should avoid actions that reward pain behavior, such as keeping the child home from school. This message should also be conveyed to others involved in the care of the child, including school authorities.

Also use "active listening" to encourage the parents and child to express their fears and concerns about how their life has been affected. Parents should be told that the child can experience increased anxiety associated with the pain, but this is no different than the anxiety experienced by other children with chronic pain. Suggest ways for the family to modify the child's environment to decrease stress. If the pain persists or if family relationships involve complex psychosocial issues, then psychological referral is indicated. A trained counselor can educate the child in how to cope with the stress associated with chronic pain and teach the parents how to manage pain behavior.

SUGGESTED READINGS

Apley J. *The child with abdominal pains*. Oxford: Blackwell Scientific Publications; 1975;3–70,71,72–104,105,106–107.

Boyle JT. Recurrent abdominal pain: an update. *Pediatr Rev* 1997;18:310–320.

Chong SKF, Lou Q, Asnicar MA, et al. *Helicobacter pylori* infection in recurrent abdominal pain in childhood: comparison of diagnostic tests and therapy. *Pediatrics* 1995; 96:211–215.

Dern MS, Stein MT. "He keeps getting stomachaches, Doctor. What's wrong?" *Contemporary Pediatrics* 1999;16:43–54.

Klish WJ. Chronic recurrent abdominal pain. In: McMillan JA, ed. *Oski's pediatrics: principles and practice*, 3rd ed. Philadelphia: Lippincott Williams & Wilkins; 1999: 1685–1686.

Lake, AM. Chronic abdominal pain in childhood: diagnosis and management. *Am Fam Physician* 1999;59:1823–1830.

Propulsid and Reglan. *Physicians' Desk Reference*, 54th ed. Montvale, NJ: Medical Economics Company, Inc., 2000: 1451–1453, 2603–2605.

Scharff L. Recurrent abdominal pain in children: a review of psychological factors and treatment. *Clin Psychol Rev* 1997;17:145–166.

Walker LS, Guite JW, Duke M, et al. Recurrent abdominal pain: a potential precursor of irritable bowel syndrome in adolescents and young adults. *J Pediatr* 1998;132: 1010–1015.

CHAPTER 3

....

Jaundice in Adults

Jory A. Natkin and Martin S. Lipsky

DEFINITION

Jaundice, also referred to as icterus, is a syndrome characterized by hyperbilirubinemia and the deposition of bile pigment in the skin, mucous membranes, and sclera that results in a yellowish appearance. Usually bilirubin levels need to be greater than 2.5 to 3.0 mg/dl for jaundice to be visible. Two major types of jaundice occur: unconjugated hyperbilirubinemia and conjugated hyperbilirubinemia. This is determined by whether the excess bilirubin (unconjugated bilirubin) has been converted to a water-soluble, or conjugated, form by the liver. The causes of jaundice can also be grouped anatomically: prehepatic, hepatic caused by hepatocellular dysfunction, and posthepatic where bilirubin excretion is impaired. Some clinicians also use the terms "obstructive jaundice" if an anatomic obstruction can be demonstrated that blocks the excretion of bilirubin and "cholestatic jaundice" in cases of an obstructive enzyme pattern but the impaired secretion is on a functional basis. However, because distinguishing between these two entities by clinical and biochemical criteria is often difficult, many times clinicians use the two terms interchangeably.

Unconjugated hyperbilirubinemia is typically present in prehepatic disease, Gilbert's syndrome, hemolysis, and the Crigler-Najjar syndrome. Conjugated hyperbilirubinemia is present in most posthepatic diseases, Dubin-Johnson and Rotor's syndromes, and most intrahepatic causes of hyperbilirubinemia.

CLINICAL MANIFESTATIONS

Because jaundice usually causes anxiety in patients, most individuals will seek prompt medical attention. Jaundiced individuals may appear ill or may look healthy except for the jaundice. Common nonspecific symptoms associated with jaundice include pruritus, nausea and vomiting, anorexia, and malaise. Dark-colored urine and light or clay-colored stools indicate an obstructive process, but they do not distinguish between obstruction related to an intrahepatic cause (e.g, viral hepatitis) and an extrahepatic cause (e.g., an underlying malignancy).

A patient experiencing abdominal pain is more likely to have an obstructive cause. For example, acute right upper quadrant pain suggests biliary tract obstruction. Age is an important variable because patients aged less than 30 years are more likely to have acute parenchymal disease, whereas patients aged more than 65 years are more likely to have an extrahepatic obstruction or malignancy. Obstruction from malignancy (e.g., pancreatic cancer) should always be considered in older patients with significant weight loss and anorexia. Chronic liver disease is most common in middle-aged individuals.

PATIENT HISTORY

Fever, arthralgias, and rash point to viral hepatitis, particularly in the presence of risk factors for hepatitis. These risk factors include exposure to hepatitis, travel to an endemic area, tattoos, intravenous (IV) drug use, and high-risk sexual practices.

Asking the patient about alcohol consumption and toxin exposure, and carefully reviewing all medications are essential. Drugs that cause intrahepatic cholestasis include estrogens and phenothiazines. Table 3.1 lists other drugs that have been associated with hyperbilirubinemia. A family history of episodic jaundice, particularly during periods of fasting or during an intercurrent viral illness, is suggestive of Gilbert's disease.

PHYSICAL EXAMINATION

A physical examination can be helpful in determining the cause and directing the evaluation of jaundice. Fever can be present in acute hepatitis, cholecystitis and cholangitis. Findings, such as a small liver, ascites, splenomegaly, spider angiomas,

T ABLE 3.1.   Common drugs associated with hyperbilirubinemia

Hepatocellular causes	Cholestatic Causes		Mixed causes
Acetaminophen	Amitriptyline	5-Flucytosine	Acetohexamide
Alcohol	Androgenic steroids (B)	Fluoroquinolones	Allopurinol
Amiodarone	Atenolol	Griseofulvin	Ampicillin
Azulfidine	Augmentin	Haloperidol (D)	Augmentin
Carbenicillin	Azathioprine	Labetalol	Cimetidine
Clindamycin	Bactrim (D)	Nicotinic acid	Dapsone
Colchicine	Benzodiazepines	NSAIDs	Disulfiram
Cyclophosphamide	Captopril	Penicillins	Gold
Diltiazem		Phenobarbital	Hydralazine
Ketoconazole	Chlordiazepoxide (D)	Phenothiazines (D)	Lovostatin
Methyldopa	Clofibrate	Phenytoin	Nitrofurantoin
Niacin	Coumadin	Tamoxifen	NSAIDs
Nifedipine	Cyclosporine	Tegretol	Phenytoin
NSAIDs	Danazol (B)	Thiabendazole (D)	Rifampin
Propylthiouracil	Dapsone	Thiazides	Sulfonamides
Pyridium	Disopyramide	Thiouracil	Tetracycline
Pyrazinamide	Erythromycin	Tolbutamide (D)	
Quinidine	Estrogens (B)	Tricyclics (D)	
Rifampin	Ethambutol	Verapamil	
Salicylates	Floxuridine	Zidovudine	
Verapamil			

B, bland or noninflammatory cholestasis; D, ductopenic cholestasis or vanishing bile duct syndrome; NSAID, non-steroidal antiinflammatory drug.

From Caldwell LA, Peters MG. Approach to the patient with jaundice. In: Yamada T, Alpers DH, Laine L, Owyang C, Powell DW, eds. *Textbook of gastroenterology*, 3rd ed. Philadelphia: Lippincott Williams & Wilkins, 1999:938.

gynecomastia, palmar erythema, and other stigmata of cirrhosis suggest advanced hepatocellular disease. Viral hepatitis usually causes a mildly tender liver with slight to moderate enlargement. Needle tracks are seen in IV drug users, and may provide a clue for hepatitis. Right upper quadrant tenderness is seen with cholecystitis and extrahepatic biliary obstruction. Although rare, Courvoisier's sign, which is a painless palpable gallbladder, suggests malignant obstruction of the common bile duct. A markedly enlarged liver is most commonly seen in metastatic cancer to the liver, severe passive congestion, and advanced infiltrative disease of the liver.

DIAGNOSTIC STUDIES

Studies can be divided into laboratory testing and imaging. Testing usually begins with a urinalysis and a liver panel test, including transaminases, total bilirubin, alkaline phosphatase, and albumin. A dipstick urine test is inexpensive and can be done quickly in the office. Because conjugated bilirubin appears in the urine, its presence suggests either obstruction, cholestasis, or hepatocellular injury. Urine negative for bilirubin in a jaundiced individual implies excessive bilirubin production or impaired conjugation. Serum levels of direct (conjugated) and indirect (unconjugated) bilirubin can confirm the urine results. Hemolysis, ineffective hematopoiesis, or a hereditary cause of jaundice are the leading causes of unconjugated hyperbilirubinemia. A reticulocyte count, lactate dehydrogenase, peripheral smear, and haptoglobin provide evidence of hemolysis and are indicated in patients with unconjugated hyperbilirubinemia.

Hepatocellular enzymes (aspartate aminotransferase and alanine aminotransferase) that are elevated out of proportion (> 5× normal) to the alkaline phosphatase (2-3× normal) suggest hepatocellular dysfunction. Conversely, an obstructive enzyme pattern is characterized by an elevated alkaline phosphatase (> 3× normal) out of proportion to the rise in hepatocellular enzymes (< 4-5× normal). Gamma glutamyl transpeptidase usually parallels the rise in alkaline phosphatase. This test is useful for confirming that an elevated alkaline phosphatase is caused by liver disease since an increase in alkaline phosphatase can also occur in bone disease.

Imaging is useful in evaluating patients for obstructive disease. Ultrasound is a noninvasive and relatively inexpensive test for detecting dilated bile ducts indicative of biliary obstruction. The sensitivity and specificity of this test is in the 85% to 95% range. Limitations include its dependence on operator technique and the difficulty in obtaining a good examination in obese patients and in those with bowel gas overlying the pancreas.

Although ultrasound can detect obstruction, it is less helpful in determining the site and cause of the obstruction. A computed tomography (CT) scan is more likely to identify the site or cause of obstruction. A CT scan has the disadvantage of being more expensive than ultrasound and entailing radiation exposure.

If an obstruction is identified and additional anatomic detail is needed, endoscopic retrograde cholangiopancreatography (ERCP) or percutaneous transhepatic cholangiography (PTC) can provide direct visualization. This test can also be useful if obstructive jaundice is strongly suspected on clinical grounds despite a negative imaging procedure. Advantages of ERCP are its ability to provide direct inspection of the upper gastrointestinal tract and Vater's ampulla. It also enables the endoscopist to obtain biopsy material and to intervene therapeutically in appropriate situations such as removing a stone trapped in the common bile duct. Complications of ERCP include infection and pancreatitis. PTC, an alternative to ERCP, allows visualization via a direct transhepatic ductal puncture. Depending on the operator's expertise, PTC is sometimes preferred in patients with previous bile duct surgery or in cases of a suspected proximal obstruction. PTC has similar risks for complications to ERCP. Magnetic resonance cholangiopancreatography (MRCP) is a newer technique that can be helpful.

RISK FACTORS

Many risk factors exist for the various disorders causing jaundice. Risk factors for viral hepatitis include multiple sexual partners, IV drug use, travel to endemic areas, and prior blood transfusions. Family history may be an important risk factor in developing alcohol dependency and its associated liver disease. It is also a factor in familial disorders such as Gilbert's syndrome or hemachromatosis. Dubin-Johnson syndrome and Rotor's syndrome are both inherited in an autosomal recessive fashion and there may be a family history of one of these disorders. Patients on multiple medications are also at risk for developing jaundice.

PATHOPHYSIOLOGY

The pathophysiology for jaundice can be divided into the following mechanisms: excess bilirubin production, decreased hepatic uptake, impaired conjugation or decreased biliary secretion, intrahepatic cholestasis, and obstructive disease. Excessive bilirubin production usually results from increased red blood cell destruction.

Decreased uptake and conjugation causes an unconjugated hyperbilirubinemia. Hereditary conditions such as Gilbert's or Crigler-Najjar syndromes are common causes. Intrahepatic cholestasis can occur at the level of the hepatocyte or bile duct. The increased bilirubin is conjugated and is usually associated with a marked increase in alkaline phosphatase. Extrahepatic obstruction occurs from a mechanical blockage from a stone, stricture, or tumor. Hepatocellular disease is typified by viral hepatitis.

DIFFERENTIAL DIAGNOSIS

Table 3.2 lists the differential diagnosis. Usually a combination of history, physical examination, and routine laboratory tests allows differentiation of obstructive from nonobstructive jaundice. For example, a history of IV drug abuse increases the risk for viral hepatitis, which can be rapidly confirmed by serology (Chapter 5). Initial laboratory studies should include a complete blood count, total and direct bilirubin, urinalysis, and liver enzymes. If unconjugated bilirubin is present, the two most likely causes are hemolysis and Gilbert's syndrome. A peripheral smear with lactate dehydrogenase, haptoglobin, and reticulocyte count will detect hemolysis. Gilbert's syndrome is characterized by recurrent mild elevations of bilirubin (1.5–3 mg/dl) often precipitated by fasting or mild illness. Patients with Gilbert's syndrome generally have no systemic symptoms and no other liver test abnormalities. Although not necessary for diagnosis, a liver biopsy in a patient with Gilbert's syndrome is normal.

Type I and type II Crigler-Najjar syndromes are rare inherited defects in bilirubin conjugation. Type I is associated with very high levels of bilirubin and death in early infancy. Type II Crigler-Najjar syndrome is associated with lower levels of bilirubin and typically has less severe clinical sequelae.

When the initial assessment suggests obstruction, an imaging study (e.g., ultrasound) is indicated. Ultrasound is technically difficult in obese patients and in those with overlying gas. For these patients and those at high risk for malignancy, a CT scan may be a better initial study. If the enzyme pattern is mixed or cirrhosis is a consideration, evaluation for illnesses such as viral hepatitis, hemachromatosis, Wilson's disease, and autoimmune hepatitis is indicated (see Chapter 5 on elevated liver enzymes). A liver biopsy may be necessary to detect infiltrative disease such as sarcoidosis, amyloidosis, or metastatic disease.

The hereditary defects of biliary excretion include Dubin-Johnson syndrome and Rotor's syndrome. Both entities usually present in childhood or adolescence. Dubin-Johnson syndrome is usually characterized by a chronic mild conjugated hyperbiliru-

T ABLE 3.2.   Differential diagnosis of adult jaundice

UNCONJUGATED HYPERBILIRUBINEMIA
Hemolysis
Defects in bilirubin conjugation
    Gilbert's syndrome
    Crigler-Najjar syndrome (I and II)
Bilirubin overproduction
    Large hematoma
    Pulmonary embolism
    Ineffective erythropoiesis

CONJUGATED HYPERBILIRUBINEMIA
Hepatocellular injury from any cause
    Medications
    Viral hepatitis
    Ethanol abuse
Cholestatic conditions, intra- and extrahepatic
    Biliary disease
    Stones
    Strictures
    Sclerosing cholangitis
    Cholangiocarcinoma
Pancreatic disease
Primary biliary cirrhosis
Metastatic cancer
Sepsis
Drug-induced cholestasis
Infiltrative liver disease
Congenital causes
    Dubin-Johnson syndrome
    Rotor's syndrome

binemia with an otherwise normal chemical profile. Occasionally, the liver can be mildly enlarged or patients have vague constitutional symptoms. A cholecystogram usually fails to visualize the gallbladder. Diagnosis can be confirmed by laparoscopy and needle biopsy. Typically, the liver is a black-brown color and hepatocytes demonstrate increased pigment.

Rotor's syndrome is clinically similar to Dubin-Johnson syndrome. However, by contrast, an oral cholecystogram typically does visualize the gallbladder and both the liver and biopsy specimens appear normal-colored.

If the liver enzymes suggest hepatocellular disease, studies such as viral serology for hepatitis, iron studies, an antismooth muscle antibody titer, and antimitochondrial antibodies may be helpful. A liver biopsy may be required for definitive diagnosis.

REFERRAL

The family physician can manage many conditions (e.g., viral hepatitis) that cause jaundice. Most patients can be treated in the outpatient setting unless evidence is seen of severe disease, dehydration, or obstructive jaundice accompanied by fever, chills, or peritoneal signs. Along with IV antibiotics, surgical consultation is indicated in febrile patients with obstructive jaundice.

Consultation with a gastroenterologist is appropriate when ERCP is indicated, in patients presenting diagnostic dilemmas, or when a liver biopsy is required for definitive diagnosis. A hematologic consultation is desirable in patients with hemolysis. Surgical consultation, along with an oncology evaluation, is necessary in most patients with neoplasm.

MANAGEMENT

The treatment of jaundice depends on its cause. If liver damage is caused by toxins (e.g., drugs or other substances), these agents need to be identified and stopped. Supportive care is indicated while monitoring the patient to assess that the liver function returns to normal. Patients with pruritus caused by marked elevations of bilirubin may benefit from bile sequestering agents, such as cholestyramine (Questran). One packet (4 g) taken 1–3 times a day usually reduces symptoms. If needed, an oral antihistamine can provide additional relief. Ancillary treatments, such as moisturizing creams and avoiding harsh soaps, sometimes provide relief. Other treatments for pruritus in liver disease are outlined in Table 3.3.

T ABLE 3.3.   Treatment of pruritus in liver disease

Decrease water temperature and increase frequency of shower or bath.

Use moisturizing soaps; avoid deodorant soaps.

Use moisturizing cream after shower or bath.

Use fewer/lighter clothes and blankets at night.

Cholestyramine (Questran) powder, 1 scoop/packet to 6 scoops/packets daily. This basic polystyrene resin binds bile salts and other factors in the gut associated with pruritus.

Ursodeoxycholic acid (Actigall), 300–900 mg/d. The mechanism may be related to the modification of the bile salt composition.

Doxepin (Sinequan), 25–50 mg daily, or other tricyclics, noting caution for symptoms of drowsiness. The mechanism of this and other similar medicines may be CNS-mediated effects or mast cell function.

Antihistamines, such as diphenhydramine (Benadryl), should be used only with extreme caution, as for the associated drowsiness and precipitation of hepatic encephalopathy in patients with chronic liver disease.

Rifampin, 300–600 mg/d. Rifampin lowers hepatocyte bile salt concentration via competitive uptake with bile salts. Liver function tests may be altered by this medicine.

Naloxone (Narcan), 0.2 mg/kg/min over 24 h. This opiate antagonist can be used for several refractory cases of pruritus, with the rationale of treating CNS opioid-mediated pruritus.

CNS, central nervous system.

From Caldwell CA, Peters MG. Approach to the patient with jaundice. In: Yamada T, Alpers DH, Laine L, Owyang C, Powell DW, eds. *Textbook of gastroenterology*, 3rd ed. Philadelphia: Lippincott Williams & Wilkins, 1999:940.

When obstruction is the cause of jaundice, surgery may be needed. For patients with cholelithiasis, either open or laparoscopic cholecystectomy is indicated. ERCP or MRCP can be valuable, both diagnostically and therapeutically. Endoscopic sphincterotomy and stone extraction may be beneficial in patients who are not surgical candidates. Surgical treatment is generally helpful for most patients with obstructive jaundice from neoplasm. This surgery can either be palliative or for definitive treatment. Procedures range from T-tube insertion to divert the flow of bile to a Whipple's procedure for pancreatic carcinoma. Input from both medical and radiation oncology and the treatment options they offer may be beneficial in many cases. In some patients, liver transplantation may be the only option.

Gilbert's syndrome is almost always benign and treatment consists of reassurance and avoiding unnecessary testing.

The management of hepatitis is outlined in Chapter 5.

Dubin-Johnson syndrome is also usually asymptomatic, although vague abdominal pain and weakness can occasionally occur. Patients with Rotor's syndrome typically also require no treatment.

Patient Education

Patients with jaundice should be advised of their condition. Those with benign hereditary conditions need to be assured that their condition is neither serious nor contagious. However, they should be aware that other family members are at risk for having the syndrome.

Patients with underlying liver disease should avoid alcohol or medications that can adversely affect their liver function. They should be immunized against viral hepatitis to avoid concomitant illness that may worsen their condition.

SUGGESTED READING

Richter JM. Evaluation of jaundice. In: Goroll AH, May LA, Mully AG Jr. *Primary Care Medicine: Office evaluation and management of the adult patient.* 3rd ed. Philadelphia: Lippincott Williams & Wilkins 1995:348–352.

Sekijima J. Jaundice. In: Fihn SD, DeWitt DE, eds. *Outpatient medicine.* Philadelphia: WB Saunders, 1998:298–302.

Ventura E. Jaundice. In: Porro GB, ed. *Gastroenterology and hepatology.* New York: McGraw-Hill, 1999:54–64.

CHAPTER 4

··

Neonatal Jaundice

Diane J. Madlon-Kay

DEFINITION

Jaundice is a yellow appearance of the skin secondary to increased concentrations of serum bilirubin. A more detailed definition is given in Chapter 3.

CLINICAL MANIFESTATIONS

Jaundice can be present at birth, and can appear at any time during the neonatal period. Jaundice typically begins in the face and, as the serum bilirubin level increases, progresses to the abdomen and feet. Infants with physiologic jaundice usually appear well. Infants with jaundice caused by hemolytic disease, sepsis, or galactosemia often have other clinical signs of illness. The challenge for family physicians is to differentiate between physiologic jaundice, seen in 60% of newborns during the first week of life, and pathologic jaundice, which may be the harbinger of a more serious condition. Diagnosis and management of jaundice has become more difficult because of the resurgence of breast-feeding, which increases the incidence of jaundice, and early hospital discharge, which occurs before the bilirubin level has peaked.

PATIENT HISTORY

The newborn's feeding history can provide clues to several possible causes of jaundice. Breast-feeding is associated with higher levels of unconjugated bilirubin and a longer duration of jaundice compared with formula-feeding. Vomiting and jaundice are seen in metabolic diseases such as galactosemia when infants are fed either breast milk or a lactose-containing formula. Vomiting can also suggest sepsis or pyloric stenosis. Both of these conditions are associated with hyperbilirubinemia.

A delayed passage of meconium or infrequent stools, which can be secondary to cystic fibrosis or Hirschsprung's disease, can lead to increased enterohepatic circulation of bilirubin. A history of pale stools and dark urine may indicate a disorder producing cholestasis.

Premature infants are susceptible to higher bilirubin levels and more prolonged hyperbilirubinemia. For each week of gestation less than 40 weeks, the risk of hyperbilirubinemia increases. In one study, infants at 37 weeks' gestation were four times more likely to have a bilirubin level = 13 mg/dl (222.3 μmol/L) than were those at 40 weeks' gestation. Premature infants are more likely to have delayed enteral feedings, require parenteral nutrition, and have perinatal insults with hypoxia and acidosis. It is particularly important to pay attention to slightly premature breast-feeding infants. Infants at 36 to 37 weeks' gestation do not nurse as well as more mature babies and need more careful follow-up.

The infant's age at onset and the duration of jaundice are also important parts of the history. The presence of jaundice within 24 hours of birth is generally considered pathologic and requires evaluation for possible hemolytic disease or other diagnoses. Jaundice persisting beyond 3 weeks also requires further evaluation.

PHYSICAL EXAMINATION

With increasing levels of bilirubin, neonatal jaundice becomes more extensive, spreading in a cephalocaudal direction. When the serum bilirubin level is approximately 6 mg/dl (102.6 µmol/L), only the head and neck are icteric. As the bilirubin increases, the jaundice extends as follows: trunk to umbilicus (bilirubin level of 9 mg/dl [153.9 µmol/L]); groin, including upper thighs (12 mg/dl [205.2 µmol/L]); knees to ankles (15 mg/dl [256.5 µmol/L]); feet, including soles (> 15 mg/dl [256.5 µmol/L]).

Infants who are small for their gestational age are frequently polycythemic and jaundiced. They may also have been exposed to an intrauterine infection. Microcephaly is seen in patients with intrauterine infections associated with jaundice. A cephalhematoma may be seen and can cause jaundice. Petechiae suggest congenital infection, sepsis, or severe hemolytic disease as a cause of the jaundice. Chorioretinitis suggests a congenital infection. Jaundice occurs more frequently in infants who have congenital anomalies from trisomic conditions. Pallor or hepatosplenomegaly suggests possible hemolytic disease.

Signs and symptoms of kernicterus, the neurologic syndrome resulting from the deposition of unconjugated bilirubin in brain cells, usually appear 2 to 5 days after birth in full-term infants. Lethargy, poor feeding, and the loss of the Moro's reflex are common initial signs. Subsequently, the infant may appear gravely ill and lethargic with diminished tendon reflexes and respiratory distress. Opisthotonos (an arched position of the body with feet and head on the floor), with bulging fontanel, twitching of face or limbs, and a shrill high-pitched cry may follow. Kernicterus is rare in healthy full-term infants and in the absence of hemolysis if the serum bilirubin level is under 25 mg/dl (427.5 µmol/L).

DIAGNOSTIC STUDIES

Maternal prenatal testing should include ABO and Rh typing and serum screening for unusual isoimmune antibodies. A direct Coombs' test, a blood type, and an Rh type on the infant's cord blood are recommended when the mother has not had prenatal blood grouping or is Rh-negative. Cord blood of all infants should be routinely saved for future testing, particularly when the mother's blood type is group O.

When family history, ethnic or geographic origin, or the timing of the appearance of jaundice suggest the possibility of glucose-6-phosphate dehydrogenase (G6PD) deficiency or some other cause of hemolytic disease, appropriate laboratory tests should be performed. Such testing should include a complete blood cell count with differential, smear, reticulocyte count, G6PD screen, and hemoglobin electrophoresis. Unfortunately, the complete blood count, reticulocyte count, and blood smear are tests with poor sensitivity and specificity for hemolysis. They are often abnormal in infants with no evidence of hemolysis or normal in hemolyzing infants. Moreover, even in large teaching hospitals, G6PD measurements are often done only twice a week.

The total serum bilirubin level should be determined in all infants noted to have jaundice in the first 24 hours of life. Infants older than 24 hours should have total serum bilirubin levels determined if the jaundice is judged to be clinically significant. An assessment of the level of cephalocaudal progression of jaundice can be helpful in determining whether to obtain a bilirubin test. Alternatively, an icterometer or

T ABLE 4.1.   Strategies for evaluation of jaundiced term infants

Maneuver	Indications
Blood type and group	All mothers
Follow infant for significant jaundice	All infants
Measure serum bilirubin level	All infants with significant jaundice
Blood type, group, Coombs' test	Total serum bilirubin level >14–15 mg/dl (239.4 to 256.5 µmol/L) and group O or Rh-negative mother
Follow bilirubin level until peak	Infants with evidence of hemolysis
Complete blood cell count or hemoglobin level	Suspicion of hemolytic disease or anemia (e.g., early jaundice or total serum bilirubin >14 mg/dl (239.4 µmol/L) in first 48 h
Reticulocyte count, blood smear	Questionable value; consider if infant is anemic or with a strong clinical suspicion of hemolytic disease other than isoimmunization
Glucose-6-phosphate dehydrogenase screen	Consider in Asian or Mediterranean infants (especially males) with total serum bilirubin level >15 mg/dl (256.5 µmol/L), particularly if late-onset jaundice
Direct bilirubin level and/or urine dipstick for bilirubin	Persistent jaundice (>2 wk) or baby ill

transcutaneous jaundice meter may be helpful in determining which infants should have bilirubin testing.

Measurements of direct bilirubin, which represents the conjugated portion, vary substantially as a result of individual laboratories and their instruments. For the purpose of the otherwise healthy-appearing newborn with jaundice, the direct bilirubin measurement should not be subtracted from the total serum bilirubin level, and the total serum bilirubin level should be relied on as the relevant criterion for determining treatment.

Approximately one third of healthy breast-fed infants have persistent jaundice after 2 weeks of age. Infants with dark urine or light stools should have a direct serum bilirubin measurement. Infants without this history can continue to be observed. If jaundice persists beyond 3 weeks, a urine sample should be tested for bilirubin, and a measurement of total and direct serum bilirubin obtained.

Evaluation of newborn infants who develop abnormal signs such as feeding difficulty, behavior changes, apnea, or temperature instability, is recommended to rule out an underlying illness, regardless of the presence of jaundice. Strategies for laboratory evaluation of jaundiced infants are summarized in Table 4.1.

RISK FACTORS

The prenatal and perinatal history may reveal several risk factors for jaundice. A family history of a parent or sibling with jaundice or anemia suggests a hereditary hemolytic anemia. If a previous sibling had a bilirubin level greater than 12 mg/dl (205.2 µmol/L), the risk of this infant having a similar bilirubin level is three times greater than that of infants whose siblings did not have that degree of jaundice as infants. If the previous sibling had a bilirubin level of 15 mg/dl (256.5 µmol/L), the risk of a similar level in this infant is increased 12 times.

A maternal history of prenatal infections (e.g., rubella, cytomegalovirus, or syphilis) may indicate jaundice caused by cholestatic liver disease. Women who smoke at least one pack of cigarettes per day during pregnancy have a lower risk of having a child with hyperbilirubinemia than those who smoke less. An increased incidence of jaundice is seen in infants of diabetic mothers because of their increased red blood cell mass. Maternal ingestion of a sulfonamide, a nitrofurantoin, or an antimalarial may initiate hemolysis in G6PD-deficient infants.

The labor and delivery history may reveal that the infant was delivered by vacuum extraction, which may have caused a cephalhematoma. Oxytocin (Pitocin) use is also associated with an increased incidence of neonatal jaundice. Delayed cord clamping can lead to polycythemia and jaundice. Infants with low Apgar scores, indicating asphyxia, have an increased incidence of jaundice.

The most important factors to consider in the history and physical examination when evaluating an infant with jaundice are summarized in Table 4.2.

East-Asian infants are much more likely to experience jaundice than are white or African-American infants. Male infants are more likely to experience jaundice than are female infants. People of Mediterranean, Nigerian, and Chinese descent, as well as Sephardic Jews, have higher frequencies of G6PD deficiency. Jaundice from G6PD deficiency tends to be of slightly later onset, at days 3 to 5 of life instead of days 2 to

T ABLE 4.2. Factors to be considered when assessing a jaundiced infant

Factors that suggest the possibility of hemolytic disease
  Family history of significant hemolytic disease
  Onset of jaundice before age 24 h
  A rise in serum bilirubin levels of more than 0.5 mg/dl per hour
  Pallor, hepatosplenomegaly
  Rapid increase in the TSB level after 24–48 h (consider G6PD deficiency)
  Ethnicity suggestive of inherited disease (e.g., G6PD deficiency)
  Failure of phototherapy to lower the TSB level
Clinical signs suggesting the possibility of other diseases such as sepsis or galactosemia in which jaundice may be one manifestation of the disease
  Vomiting
  Lethargy
  Poor feeding
  Hepatosplenomegaly
  Excessive weight loss
  Apnea
  Temperature instability
  Tachypnea
Signs of cholestatic jaundice suggesting the need to rule out biliary atresia or other causes of cholestasis
  Dark urine or urine positive for bilirubin
  Light-colored stools
  Persistent jaundice for >3 wk

G6PD, glucose-6-phosphate dehydrogenase; TSB, total serum bilirubin.

Reprinted from Practice parameter: management of hyperbilirubinemia in the healthy term newborn. *Pediatrics* 1994;94:559; with permission.

3. A history of a previous sibling with neonatal jaundice suggests hemolytic disease caused by ABO or Rh isoimmunization, or breast milk jaundice.

PATHOPHYSIOLOGY

The newborn infant's metabolism of bilirubin is in transition from the fetal stage (when the placenta is the principal route of elimination of bilirubin) to the adult stage. The mature liver maintains relatively stable nontoxic concentrations of bilirubin in the blood and tissues such as the brain. Bilirubin is derived from the breakdown of heme. Free (unbound to plasma protein), unconjugated bilirubin is a potential neurotoxin. After binding to albumin in the systemic circulation, bilirubin is transported to the liver. The liver converts bilirubin to its conjugated form. Conjugated bilirubin is then excreted in the feces, where a variable portion may be reabsorbed.

Several factors lead to a mild degree of jaundice in most infants in the first days of life: (a) increased hemolysis from trauma inherent in the birth process; (b) immature uptake or conjugation in the liver; and (c) enterohepatic recirculation of bilirubin. Disease processes can interrupt bilirubin metabolism at any step in the pathway and, thereby, predispose an infant to kernicterus.

DIFFERENTIAL DIAGNOSIS

The differential diagnosis is outlined in Tables 4.3 and 4.4.

REFERRAL

Family physicians can safely and effectively evaluate and treat, without consultation, most healthy full-term, jaundiced infants. Consultation with a pediatrician or neonatologist should be considered for the following infants: premature infants, infants with cholestatic jaundice, ill-appearing infants, infants whose bilirubin levels fail to respond to intensive phototherapy, and infants requiring exchange transfusions.

MANAGEMENT

Management of jaundice depends on the cause. The management of jaundice caused by conjugated hyperbilirubinemia usually requires referral and is beyond the scope of this chapter. Similarly, the management of jaundice in premature infants or otherwise ill infants cannot be adequately discussed in this chapter.

The American Academy of Pediatrics' guidelines for the use of phototherapy and exchange transfusion in healthy term newborns are shown in Table 4.5. Infants aged 24 or fewer hours are excluded from Table 4.5 because jaundice occurring at this age is generally considered pathologic and requires further evaluation. Phototherapy or exchange transfusion may be indicated for rapidly rising bilirubin levels in the first 24 hours of life.

No standardized method exists for delivering phototherapy. Phototherapy units vary widely, as do the types of lamps used. Phototherapy efficiency is improved by increasing the surface area of skin exposed to the lights. This can be done by placing the infant on a fiberoptic blanket while using a standard phototherapy system. If fiberoptic units are not available, several phototherapy lamps can be placed around the infant. The area of exposure can also be increased by removing the baby's diaper and placing a white reflecting surface (e.g., a sheet) around the bassinet so that light is reflected onto the baby's skin. It is impossible to "overdose" the patient with the light sources commonly used.

T ABLE 4.3.   Differential diagnosis of unconjugated hyperbilirubinemia in infants

INCREASED BILIRUBIN PRODUCTION

Isoimmunization
  Rh incompatibility
  ABO incompatibility
  Minor blood group incompatibility
Congenital spherocytosis
Hereditary elliptocytosis
Infantile pyknocytosis
Erythrocyte enzyme defects
  G6PD
  Pyruvate kinase
  Hexokinase
Infection
Extravascular blood
  Cephalhematoma
  Intraventricular bleeding
  Bruising

Occult hematoma (renal, hepatic, adrenal,
  pulmonary, subdural)
Hemangioma
Swallowed maternal blood
Polycythemia
  Diabetic mother
  Fetal transfusion (maternal, twin)
  Delayed cord clamping
  Intrauterine growth retardation
Drugs
  Vitamin K
  Maternal oxytocin
  Phenol disinfectants
Total parenteral nutrition
Hemoglobin chain abnormalities
Disseminated intravascular coagulopathy

DECREASED BILIRUBIN UPTAKE, STORAGE, OR METABOLISM

Crigler-Najjar (I or II) syndrome
Gilbert's syndrome
Lucey-Driscoll syndrome
Drug inhibition
Hypothyroidism or hypopituitarism
Congestive heart failure
Portacaval shunt
Hypoxia
Acidosis
Sepsis

ENTEROHEPATIC RECIRCULATION

Breast milk jaundice
Intestinal obstruction
  Ileal atresia
  Hirschsprung's disease
  Cystic fibrosis
  Pyloric stenosis
Antibiotic administration

G6PD, glucose-6-phosphate dehydrogenase.

T ABLE 4.4. Differential diagnosis of conjugated hyperbilirubinemia in infants

EXTRAHEPATIC BILIARY DISEASE
Extrahepatic biliary atresia
Choledochal cyst
Bile-duct stenosis
Spontaneous perforation of the bile duct
Neoplasm
Cholelithiasis

INTRAHEPATIC BILIARY DISEASE
Intrahepatic bile-duct paucity
Inspissated bile
Caroli's disease
Congenital hepatic fibrosis and infantile polycystic disease

HEPATOCELLULAR DISEASE

Metabolic and genetic disease	Hepatitis B
Disorders of amino acid metabolism (tyrosinemia)	Hepatitis C
Disorders of lipid metabolism	Varicella
Disorders of carbohydrate metabolism	Coxsackie viruses
Peroxisomal disorders	Echoviruses
Endocrine disorders	Bacterial
Familial with uncharacterized excretory defect	Sepsis
Defective bile acid synthesis	Urinary tract infection
Defective protein synthesis	Gastroenteritis
Chromosomal disorders	Listeriosis
Infectious	Iatrogenic
Viral	Total parenteral nutrition
Cytomegalovirus	Drug or toxin
Rubella	Idiopathic
Herpes	Neonatal hepatitis
Toxoplasmosis	Miscellaneous shock or hypoperfusion
Syphilis	

Intensive phototherapy should produce a decline in the total serum bilirubin of 1 to 2 mg/dl (17.1 μmol/L to 34.2 μmol/L) within 4 to 6 hours. The bilirubin should continue to fall and remain below the threshold level for exchange transfusion. If this does not occur, phototherapy is considered a failure and exchange transfusion should be performed.

Phototherapy can be interrupted during feeding or brief parental visits. Routine supplementation with dextrose water is not indicated in infants receiving phototherapy. Some infants who are admitted with high bilirubin levels may be mildly dehydrated and may require supplemental fluid intake to correct the dehydration. These infants are almost always breast-fed. The best fluid to use is a milk-based for-

T ABLE 4.5. Management of hyperbilirubinemia in the healthy term newborn

Age (h)	TSB Level, mg/dl (μmol/L)			
	Consider phototherapy[a]	Phototherapy	Exchange transfusion if intensive phototherapy fails[b]	Exchange transfusion and intensive phototherapy
≤24[c]	—	—	—	—
25–48	≥12 (170)	≥15 (260)	≥20 (340)	≥25 (430)
49–72	≥15 (260)	≥18 (310)	≥25 (430)	≥30 (510)
>72	≥17 (290)	≥20 (340)	≥25 (430)	≥30 (510)

TSB, total serum bilirubin.

[a]Phototherapy at these TSB levels is a clinical option, meaning that the intervention is available and may be used *on the basis of individual clinical judgment.*

[b]Intensive phototherapy should produce a decline of TSB of 1 to 2 mg/dl within 4 to 6 h and the TSB level should continue to fall and remain below the threshold level for exchange transfusion. If this does not occur, it is considered a failure of phototherapy.

[c]Term infants who are clinically jaundiced at ≤24 h old are not considered healthy and require further evaluation.

From Practice parameter: management of hyperbilirubinemia in the healthy term newborn. *Pediatrics* 1994;94:560; with permission.

mula because it inhibits the enterohepatic circulation of bilirubin and helps lower the serum bilirubin level.

Many studies have demonstrated that home phototherapy is safe and effective, and achieves a high degree of parental satisfaction. A fiberoptic blanket is frequently used. One of the greatest advantages of the blanket is that it facilitates the infant being held by a parent while receiving phototherapy. Eye patches are unnecessary, which means the parents can make eye contact with their infant. It is probably prudent to limit home phototherapy to full-term infants who have no signs of infection or hemolytic disease.

In infants with jaundice associated with breast-feeding, encourage continued and frequent breast-feeding, at least 8 to 10 times every 24 hours. Supplementing breast milk with plain water or dextrose water does not lower the bilirubin level in healthy, breast-feeding infants with jaundice. Less optimal options are supplementation of breast-feeding with formula, or the temporary interruption of breast-feeding and substitution with formula, either of which can be accompanied by phototherapy.

An investigational approach to the treatment of hyperbilirubinemia is the development of drugs called hemeoxygenase inhibitors, such as tin mesoporphyrin. They work by delaying the formation of bilirubin. In one study, a single intramuscular injection of one of these medications eliminated the need for phototherapy. These compounds have been found to be effective in both full-term and preterm infants, and in those with and without hemolytic disease. Research continues to be focused on optimal drug doses, clinical strategies for their use, and potential toxicity.

FOLLOW-UP

In infants who do not have hemolytic disease, the average bilirubin rebound after phototherapy is less than 1 mg/dl (< 17.1 μmol/L). Phototherapy can be discontinued when the serum bilirubin level falls below 14 to 15 mg/dl (239.4 to 256.5 µmol/L). Discharge from the hospital need not be delayed in order to observe the infant for rebound, and no further measurement of bilirubin is necessary.

Follow-up by a healthcare professional in an office, clinic, or at home should be provided within 2 to 3 days of discharge to all neonates discharged less than 48 hours after birth. One purpose of this visit is to assess the infant's degree of jaundice.

PATIENT EDUCATION

Before discharge from the hospital, the parents should be instructed how to recognize signs of jaundice. The parents should be instructed to look at the baby under natural daylight or in a room that has fluorescent lights, and to look for jaundice by gently pressing a fingertip on the tip of the baby's nose or forehead and looking at the color of the underlying skin.

Current treatments for jaundice, such as temporarily interrupting breast-feeding, and using phototherapy (which involves separation from the infant) are upsetting to mothers. Many mothers of otherwise healthy full-term infants consider jaundice a serious illness, and their concern often persists for months. Before recommending treatment for jaundice, physicians need to reassure parents that their infant is basically healthy, and to support and encourage their ability to care for minor problems.

SUGGESTED READINGS

Bland H. Jaundice in the healthy term neonate: when is treatment indicated? *Curr Probl Pediatr* 1996;26:355-363.

Lasker MR, Holzman IR. Neonatal jaundice. When to treat, when to watch and wait. *Postgrad Med* 1996;99:187-192, 197-198.

Maisels MJ. Clinical rounds in the well-baby nursery: treating jaundiced newborns. *Pediatr Ann* 1995;25:547-552.

Newman TB, Maisels MJ. Evaluation and treatment of jaundice in the term newborn: a kinder, gentler approach. *Pediatrics* 1992;89:809-818.

Provisional Committee for Quality Improvement and Subcommittee on Hyperbilirubinemia. Practice parameter: management of hyperbilirubinemia in the healthy term newborn. *Pediatrics* 1994;94:558-565.

CHAPTER 5

Elevated Liver Enzymes

Robert M. Wolfe

DEFINITION

The workup of elevated liver enzymes is a common challenge facing family physicians. Although the term "liver function test" is often used to describe liver enzyme evaluations, the term should be reserved for biochemical tests that assess the functional hepatic reserve—traditionally, the albumin level and the prothrombin time. The liver enzymes include the aminotransferases, alkaline phosphatase (ALP), and gamma-glutamyltransferase (GGT). Aminotransferases (also known as transaminases) include aspartate aminotransferase (AST, formerly known as SGOT) and alanine aminotransferase (ALT, formerly known as SGPT). Routine liver function tests screen for three functions: cellular integrity, protein synthesis, and excretory function. The aminotransferases measure cellular integrity, whereas ALP and GGT measure excretory function.

Two other enzymes, 5′-nucleotidase (5′-NT) and leucine aminopeptidase (LAP), are occasionally used for further investigation of suspected liver disease. These are discussed briefly in the *Pathophysiology* section.

CLINICAL MANIFESTATIONS

Asymptomatic Elevation of Liver Enzymes

Fatty liver, alcohol-related liver damage, and chronic viral hepatitis are the most common causes of abnormal liver function test results in asymptomatic patients. Table 5.1 summarizes findings of several studies of abnormal aminotransferase levels in asymptomatic patients. The combined results from these studies show that fatty liver (42%) and inflammation from chronic hepatitis (24%) were the most common causes of abnormal liver enzyme test results. Signs of hepatic alcohol toxicity were present in 14%. Bates and Yellin found ALP and AST elevations in 4% of approximately 5,000 people who participated in a multiphasic screening program. Fewer than 25% of patients with ALP or AST elevations eventually were given a diagnosis of liver disease. Other studies show similar results.

Liver disease can be classified as hepatocellular, cholestatic, and infiltrative (e.g., neoplasm, tuberculosis). Table 5.2 lists the frequency of occurrence of various liver diseases that cause elevations of liver enzymes.

Symptomatic Elevation of Liver Enzymes

Symptoms of anorexia, nausea, vomiting, and low-grade fever are common in patients with liver disease, but do not help much with the differential diagnosis. Symptoms of deep jaundice, pruritus, clay-colored stools, and dark-colored urine suggest cholestasis. Cholestasis is either intrahepatic (related to a defect of secretion of bile at hepatocyte level), or extrahepatic (related to structural obstruction in the biliary tree). Biliary colic, especially when associated with fever and chills, indicates that the cause of cholestasis is most likely to be in the extrahepatic biliary tree related to gallstones or tumor. Often fatigue is the only symptom of chronic liver disease. Other important general symptoms include weight loss, abdominal pain, arthralgia, itching, and rashes.

T ABLE 5.1. Prevalence of clinical and histopathologic findings in asymptomatic patients with chronically elevated aminotransferase results

Study	Magnitude of abnormality	Duration of abnormality	Exclusions	Sample size	Fatty liver	Inflammation	Alcohol-related (total)	Miscellaneous	Cirrhosis
Hultcrantz, et al.	1.5 to 10 times normal	>6 mo	Elevated alkaline phosphatase or signs and symptoms of liver disease	149	81 (54%)	31 (21%)	17 (11%)	15 (10%)	5 (3%)
Hay, et al.	3 to 8 times normal	>6 mo	Signs or symptoms of liver disease or a history of hepatitis B, transfusion, homosexuality or drug or alcohol use	47	10 (21%)	18 (38%)	N/A	3 (6%)	16 (34%)
Van Ness and Diehl	>1.5 times normal	>3 mo	Refused biopsy, previous biopsy or biopsy for staging of cancer	90	17 (19%)	28 (31%)	23 (26%)	21 (23%)	1 (1%)
Hultcrantz and Gabrielsson	Persistent elevation	>6 mo	Renal disease or signs or symptoms of liver disease	83	45 (54%)	11 (13%)	10 (12%)	3 (3%)	4 (5%)
Total				369	153 (42%)	88 (24%)	50 (14%)	42 (11%)	26 (7%)

N/A, not applicable.

Adapted from Thea RM, Scott K. Evaluating asymptomatic patients with abnormal liver function test results. *Am Fam Physician* 1996;53: 2111–2119; with permission.

T ABLE 5.2. Frequency of liver diseases

Liver Diseases	
Hepatocellular diseases[a]	**Cholestatic/infiltrative diseases**[b]
Common	**Common**
Chronic viral hepatitis	Biliary obstruction (stone, stricture, tumor)
Alcoholic liver disease	Neoplasms (metastatic, primary)
Nonalcoholic steatohepatitis	Drug hepatotoxicity (see Table 5.4)
Genetic hemochromatosis (northern European descent)	Primary biliary cirrhosis
Medication toxicity (see Table 5.4)	Primary sclerosing cholangitis
Autoimmune hepatitis	
	Less common
Less common	Autoimmune cholangiopathy
Wilson's disease	Sarcoidosis
Alpha-1 antitrypsin deficiency	

Adapted from Younossi ZM. Evaluating asymptomatic patients with mildly elevated liver enzymes. *Clev Clin J Med* 1998;65(3):150–158; with permission.

[a]Aminotransferase elevations predominate.

[b]Alkaline phosphatase and gamma-glutamyltransferase elevations predominate.

Patients with cirrhosis may present with subtle neuropsychiatric symptoms, such as lack of concentration, memory loss, and difficulty writing. Wilson's disease may present with tremor, lack of coordination, dysarthria, and behavioral changes (e.g., aggression, neuroses, psychoses).

Arthritis or arthralgias are seen in up to 25% of patients with acute hepatitis B. Arthritis usually presents with symmetric, polyarticular involvement of the proximal interphalangeal joints, knees, ankles, shoulders, and wrists. Hemochromatosis may present with arthritis of the small joints of the hand, especially the 2nd and 3rd metacarpophalangeal joints. Inflammatory bowel disease may present as spondyloarthropathy with abnormal liver function tests.

PATIENT HISTORY

When taking the medical and family history, seek clues for specific diseases. Common explanations of elevated aminotransferases include fatty liver, alcohol liver disease, chronic hepatitis B, chronic hepatitis C, and hemochromatosis. Less common explanations of elevated aminotransferase levels include drug-induced liver disease, autoimmune hepatitis, α_1-antitrypsin deficiency, Wilson's disease, hepatic granulomas, and liver tumors (Table 5.2).

Important factors are the patient's sexual history, travel, volume and duration of alcohol use, drug use, intake of vitamin A or other dietary supplements, consumption of raw oysters (hepatitis A), and history of blood transfusion or needle stick injury. Prior surgery is an important clue. Previously hospitalized patients are at increased risk for viral hepatitis.

Ask about extrahepatic illnesses, such as cardiac disease, inflammatory bowel disease, thyroid disease, and conditions of hemochromatosis, such as diabetes, skin pigmentation, cardiac disease, arthritis, and hypogonadism. Checking old medical records can help determine the chronicity of the problem. Table 5.3 lists findings from the medical history that can aid in the diagnosis of abnormal liver enzymes.

The occupational and environmental history can give important clues, such as a history of exposure to household or industrial chemicals (e.g., vinyl chloride or carbon tetrachloride).

Completely review all medications, both prescription and over-the-counter, as well as herbal products. Remedies such as germander, Jin Bu Huan anodyne tablets, and

T ABLE 5.3.   Abnormal liver function tests: history

Suggestive findings	Possible diagnoses
Acute Illness	
Fatigue, anorexia, myalgias	Acute viral hepatitis
Right upper quadrant/epigastric pain, nausea, vomiting	Acute biliary tract disease, viral hepatitis, consider HELLP syndrome if pregnant
Fever	Viral hepatitis, neoplasm, liver abscess, alcoholic hepatitis, drug-induced hepatitis, biliary tract disease
History of Blood Transfusion (check surgical history carefully)	Chronic hepatitis B, chronic hepatitis C
Alcohol History (quantitate and verify)	Alcoholic hepatitis
Drug History (Prescription drugs, OTC drugs, Drugs of abuse Vitamins (A)	Drug-induced hepatitis
Previous "hepatitis"?	Alcohol, hepatitis B, hepatitis C
Diseases and Common Predisposing Factors	
AIDS/HIV+	Hepatitis B, hepatitis C, CMV, tuberculosis
Diabetes, Obesity	Fatty liver
Congestive heart failure	Passive hepatic congestion
Inflammatory bowel disease	Common: fatty liver, pericholangitis, cholelithiasis
	Uncommon: sclerosing cholangitis, chronic hepatitis, granulomas
	Rare: amyloidosis
Pregnancy	Cholestasis of pregnancy, severe preeclampsia/HELLP syndrome, acute fatty liver of pregnancy, hyperemesis gravidarum
Other Clues	
Pruritus	Primary biliary cirrhosis, cholestasis of pregnancy
Arthritis	Hemochromatosis, hepatitis B, connective tissue disease
COPD	Alpha-1-antitrypsin deficiency, alcohol
Cardiomyopathy	Alcohol, hemochromatosis, amyloidosis, chronic passive congestion
Neuropsychiatric symptoms	Hepatic encephalopathy, Wilson's disease
Family history of liver disease	Hemochromatosis, Wilson's disease, alcoholism, chronic viral hepatitis

AIDS, acquired immunodeficiency syndrome; CMV, cytomegalovirus; COPD, chronic obstructive pulmonary disease; HELLP, hemolysis, elevated liver enzymes, low platelets; HIV, human immunodeficiency virus; OTC, over-the-counter.

From Anderson PB. Liver dysfunction. In: Reilly BM, ed. *Practical strategies in outpatient medicine*, 2nd ed. Philadelphia: WB Saunders, 1991:792; with permission.

chaparral leaf have been associated with hepatotoxicity. Some drugs and compounds that can cause hepatotoxicity are listed in Table 5.4.

Family History

A family history of severe liver disease may indicate Wilson's disease, hemochromatosis, or α_1-antitrypsin deficiency, all of which can be associated with chronic

T ABLE 5.4. Drugs and other substances that may cause abnormal liver test results

Cholestasis	Hepatocellular damage	
Antithyroid agents	Chemicals	Antihypertensive agents (continued)
Methimazole (Tapazole)	Chlorinated hydrocarbons	Diltiazem (Cardizem)
	Vinyl chloride	Captopril (Capoten)
Oral hypoglycemic agents	Arsenic	Hydralazine (Apresoline)
Glyburide (Micronase)	Benzene derivatives	Nifedipine (Procardia)
Acetohexamide (Dymelor)	Carbon tetrachloride	
Tolazamide (Tolinase)	Yellow phosphorus	Antiepileptics
		Phenytoin (Dilantin)
Antidopaminergic agents	Herbs	Carbamazepine (Tegretol)
Chlorpromazine (Thorazine)	Chaparral leaf	Valproic acid (Depacon)
Haloperidol (Haldol)	Germander	
Prochlorperazine (Compazine)	Jin Bu Huan	Antihyperlipidemic agents
Promethazine (Phenergan)	Senecio	Sustained-release niacin
	Skullcap	Clofibrate (Atromid-S)
Antibiotics	Valerian	Lovastatin (Mevacor)
Nitrofurantoin (Macrodantin)		
Erythromycin estolate	Antibiotics	Steroids
	Isoniazid (INH)	Estrogens
Histamine blockers	Griseofulvin (Grisactin)	Danazol (Danocrine)
Cimetidine (Tagamet)	Sulfonamides	
Ranitidine (Zantac)	Tetracycline	Antiarthritis agents
		Acetaminophen
Others	Antifungal agents	Piroxicam (Feldene)
Imipramine (Tofranil)	Fluconazole (Diflucan)	
Anabolic steroids	Itraconazole (Sporanox)	Others
Oral contraceptives	Ketoconazole (Nizoral)	Allopurinol (Zyloprim)
		Amiodarone (Cordarone)
	Antiviral agents	Halothane (Fluothane)
	Zidovudine (Retrovir)	Isotretinoin (Accutane)
	Didanosine (Videx)	Methotrexate
		Anti-thyroid agent
	Antihypertensive agents	Quinidine
	Methyldopa (Aldomet)	Tamoxifen (Nolvadex)
	Chlorothiazide (Diuril)	Vitamin A

Adapted from Thea RM, Scott K. Evaluating asymptomatic patients with abnormal liver function test results. *Am Fam Phys* 1996;53:2111–2119, with permission.

asymptomatic aminotransferase elevation. Hemochromatosis can also be associated with a family history of diabetes mellitus or heart failure, and α_1-antitrypsin deficiency can be associated with pulmonary emphysema.

Social History

Promiscuous sexual behavior and intravenous (IV) drug use are associated with hepatitis B and hepatitis C, and human immunodeficiency virus (HIV) infection. The patient's sexual history can also give other important clues. Estrogen contraceptives have been associated with hepatic vein thrombosis (Budd-Chiari syndrome), hepatic adenoma, and intrahepatic cholestasis. Infertility may be a presenting symptom in women with chronic active hepatitis. Pregnant women are susceptible to a variety of liver problems that can raise liver enzyme levels, including the HELLP syndrome (hemolysis, elevated liver enzymes, and low platelets), toxemia, intrahepatic cholestasis of pregnancy (IHCP), and acute fatty liver of pregnancy (AFLP).

Alcoholic liver disease may be suggested by a history of excessive alcohol ingestion (> 80–120 g/d) and is typically associated with modestly increased AST levels along with normal or minimally elevated ALT levels (increased AST:ALT ratio). Remember, patients often under-report alcohol intake. Screening tests such as the CAGE questionnaire presented in Table 5.5 may be helpful.

Review of Systems

A comprehensive review of systems is essential to uncover hepatic abnormalities that may be associated with other disorders. Diabetes mellitus, thyroid disease, congestive heart failure, collagen vascular diseases, inflammatory bowel disease, sarcoidosis, and many chronic infectious diseases can be associated with aminotransferase elevations. Table 5.6 lists a number of systemic illnesses that can manifest as hepatic disease.

PHYSICAL EXAMINATION

The physical examination can provide many clues for the patient with elevated liver enzymes. Spider angiomas, palmar erythema, and splenomegaly are typically associated with cirrhosis. Tattoos are significant as a possible source of hepatitis infection. Jaundice or scleral icterus indicates cholestasis or severe hepatocellular injury. Findings of desquamative dermatitis, cheilosis, and alopecia are associated with hepatotoxicity from hypervitaminosis A.

The abdominal examination should include liver and spleen size. Massive liver enlargement is associated with chronic passive congestion, or may be caused by tumor or fat infiltration. A nodular liver is suggestive of cirrhosis or tumor. Liver tenderness can be caused by a variety of conditions, including acute viral or alcoholic hepatitis, abscess, tumor, or acute congestion secondary to heart failure. Other signs of chronic liver injury, such as ascites, gynecomastia, testicular atrophy, abdominal venous collaterals, caput medusae, asterixis, or tremor (especially flapping tremor) should be noted.

T ABLE 5.5.   CAGE questionnaire[a]

C	Have you ever felt the need to **cut down** on your drinking?
A	Have you ever felt **angered** or **annoyed** by comments about your drinking?
G	Have you ever felt **guilty** about your drinking?
E	Do you ever have a morning **eye opener** (i.e., a drink soon after awakening)?

[a]One or more positive responses is suggestive of dependence on alcohol.

T ABLE 5.6.   Hepatic manifestations of systemic disease

Disease	Comment
Diabetes mellitus	Must distinguish fatty liver from steatohepatitis
Tuberculosis	Hepatic granulomata; typically, moderate ALP elevation only
Sarcoidosis	Hepatic granulomata; typically, moderate ALP elevation only
Amyloidosis	Hepatomegaly common
	Liver tests nonspecific
Congestive heart failure	Hepatomegaly common
	Prolonged prothrombin time especially common
Psoriasis	Hepatotoxicity due to treatment with methotrexate
Systemic lupus erythematosus	Patients especially susceptible to salicylate hepatotoxicity
Inflammatory bowel disease	Hepatic dysfunction (granulomata, chronic hepatitis, cirrhosis, pericholangitis, sclerosing cholangitis may precede onset of bowel symptoms by months or years)
Hyperthyroidism	Elevated AST and ALP levels in 45% to 90% of patients; liver function tests normalize with control of hyperthyroidism
Hypothyroidism caused by Hashimoto's thyroiditis	Increased incidence of autoimmune chronic active hepatitis and primary biliary cirrhosis
Systemic Viral Diseases with Hepatic Involvement	
Infectious mononucleosis	Liver involvement common (characteristically, atypical lymphocytosis and positive Monospot test)
Cytomegalovirus	Liver involvement common
	Most common cause of "heterophile-negative" mononucleosis
	Common in "postperfusion syndrome" after cardiopulmonary bypass
	Patients with AIDS, organ transplant especially susceptible

AIDS, acquired immune deficiency syndrome; ALP, alkaline phosphatase; AST, aminotransferase.

Clues to the diagnosis of Wilson's disease include a family history of liver disease, presence of Kayser-Fleischer rings in the cornea on slit-lamp examination (corneal limbus pigmentation), and neurologic abnormalities, especially tremor or dystonia. Hemochromatosis should be suspected in any male patient with undiagnosed chronic elevated liver enzymes. It is the most common genetic liver disease, with a homozygosity frequency of 1:220. It is associated with increased skin pigmentation and heart disease, but these are frequently absent. Examination findings in alcoholic hepatitis may include hepatomegaly, and parotid and lacrimal gland enlargement. An outline of a complete physical examination appropriate for patients with elevated liver enzymes can be found in Table 5.7.

PATHOPHYSIOLOGY

Aminotransferase elevation (ALT or AST) suggests hepatocellular damage. Normal values: < 40 U/L for AST and < 50 I/L for ALT.
- Aminotransferases include aspartate aminotransferase (AST, formerly known as SGOT) and alanine aminotransferase (ALT, formerly known as SGPT). The amino-transferases (also know as transaminases) catalyze the transfer of amino groups from aspartate and alanine, respectively, to alpha ketoglutarate. AST is found in

T ABLE 5.7. Elevated liver enzymes: physical examination

Suggestive findings	Possible diagnoses
Dermatologic Findings	
Jaundice	Hyperbilirubinemia
Gray skin	Hemochromatosis
Excoriations	Primary biliary cirrhosis
Spider angiomata, palmar erythema	Cirrhosis
Tattoos, needle tracks	Hepatitis B, hepatitis C
Evidence Suggestive of Cirrhosis	
Encephalopathy (slurred speech, forgetfulness)	
Asterixis	
Ascites, edema	
Splenomegaly	
Testicular atrophy (normal ~5 cm; atrophic ~2.5 cm)	
Caput medusae (dilated abdominal wall veins)	
Spider angiomata (on upper thorax, arms, dorsum of hands, face)	
Liver Size and Consistency	
Massively enlarged	Chronic passive congestion, tumor, fat
Mildly enlarged	Many causes
Nodular	Tumor, cirrhosis
Tender	Hepatitis (e.g., viral, alcoholic), congestive (cardiogenic), hepatomegaly, hepatic abscess, tumor
Small	Cirrhosis
Clues to Cause	
Alcohol on breath, Rhinophyma, gynecomastia, parotid and lacrimal gland enlargement	Alcohol
Tremor, ataxia, dysarthria	Wilson's disease (Kayser-Fleischer rings)
Alopecia, vitiligo	Autoimmune hepatitis
Palpable gallbladder	Carcinoma of the pancreas
Fever	Viral hepatitis, neoplasm, liver abscess, alcoholic hepatitis, drug-induced biliary tract disease
Heme-positive stool	Alcohol, colon cancer, inflammatory bowel disease

From Anderson PB, Liver Dysfunction. In: Reilly BM, ed. *Practical strategies in outpatient medicine*, 2nd ed. Philadelphia: WB Saunders, 1991:793; with permission.

heart, muscle, kidney, and brain in addition to the liver. Necrosis in any of these can elevate AST. In the cell, AST is found in both cytoplasm and mitochondria. ALT is found primarily in cytoplasm of the hepatocyte and is more specific for the liver.

Alkaline phosphatase (ALP) elevation suggests biliary obstruction, injury to the bile duct epithelium, and cholestasis. Normal values: 20 to 120 U/L.

- Alkaline phosphatase (ALP) is found in several tissues: bone, intestine, kidney, placenta, and leukocytes. ALP production tends to increase in tissues undergoing metabolic stimulation. Thus, ALP serum activity during adolescence is up to three times that of adults due to rapid bone growth and also rises during late pregnancy due to placental growth and metabolism. Cholestasis results in increased hepatic ALP synthesis, solubilization of enzyme from the biliary canalicular and sinusoidal membranes, leakage through intracellular junctions, and subsequent increased plasma enzyme activity. Any injury to the liver results in elevation of ALP, but cholestasis produces the largest elevation.

Gamma GlutamylTransferase (GGT) elevation is a marker of either type of disease, but is most sensitive to biliary tract disease. Normal values: 0 to 50 U/L in men and 0 to 35 U/L in women.

- Gamma glutamyltransferase (GGT) is a microsomal enzyme, so it is inducible, and levels are elevated by alcohol, and drugs that are strong hepatic microsomal enzyme inducers, such as phenytoin, phenobarbital, and other anticonvulsants. It has a high sensitivity for liver disorder; and abnormal activity is found in about 90% of patients with liver disease. However, specificity for liver disorders is limited by the fact that it is elevated in many other conditions that are not primarily hepatic (e.g., obesity, rheumatoid arthritis, renal failure, myocardial infarction, pancreatic disease, diabetes). Levels are reduced in pregnancy. GGT is of little value in differential diagnosis of the various liver diseases, although the highest levels (>10× upper reference limit) are found in cholestasis and hepatic malignancy. More modest elevations are found in acute and chronic hepatitis < 5× upper reference limit). GGT is most useful for confirming that an elevated ALP is of hepatobiliary origin.

Other liver enzymes

5'-nucleotidase (5'-NT) is found in hepatocyte sinusoidal and the canalicular plasma membranes, but is also present in many other tissues, such as intestine, brain, heart, and pancreas. It can be used, like GGT, to confirm the hepatobiliary origin of an elevated ALP.

Leucine-aminopeptidase (LAP) is abundant in biliary epithelium, as well as other tissues. Although it can be used to confirm the biliary origin of an elevated ALP, some authorities prefer GGT or 5'-NT for this.

DIAGNOSTIC STUDIES

Evaluation for Elevated Aspartate Aminotransferase (AST) or Alanine Aminotransferase (ALT)

The first step in the evaluation of elevated liver enzymes is to repeat the laboratory test(s). It is important to remember that most reference intervals (normal ranges) are based on the mean ± 2 standard deviations (i.e., on 95th percentile values); thus, 5% of the "normal" population will have a value for a particular test that is above or below this range. On statistical grounds alone, the likelihood of all the values on a battery of **n** tests being normal is $(0.95)^n$. For a panel of 20 tests, this means that $(0.95)^{20}$, or 64% of "normal" patients, will have at least one test outside the normal range. Thus, any isolated borderline abnormality seen should be repeated; if the abnormality persists, then the patient should be evaluated further.

In the case of an elevated AST, the AST should be repeated along with ALT testing. An isolated AST increase in the absence of an ALT increase is suggestive of cardiac or muscle disease. A rare cause of increased AST in the absence of an increase in ALT is when AST exists as a macroenzyme (macro-AST). In this condition, the AST is complexed with an immunoglobulin and, thus, is not cleared from the blood. Macro-AST does not indicate significant liver disease.

The degree of elevation of the aminotransferases can provide useful information (Table 5.8). Marked elevations, exceeding 1,000 IU/L, are suggestive of viral hepatitis, drug- or toxin-induced hepatitis, or liver ischemia. With more modest elevations

T ABLE 5.8. General patterns of liver enzyme tests[a]

Test	Hepatocellular necrosis			Biliary obstruction		Hepatic infiltration
	Toxin/ischemia	Viral	Alcohol	Complete	Partial	
	Acetaminophen or shock liver	Hepatitis A or B		Pancreatic carcinoma	Hilar tumor, primary sclerosing cholangitis	Primary or metastatic carcinoma, tuberculosis
Aminotransferase (AST, ALT)	50–100×	5–50×	2–5×	1–5×	1–5×	1–3×
Alkaline phosphatase (ALP)	1–3×	1–3×	1–10×	2–20×	2–10×	1–20×

[a]Includes illustrative disorders for each category.

From Davern TJ, Scharschmidt BF. Biochemical liver tests. In: Feldman M, ed. *Sleisenger and Fordtran's Gastrointestinal and Liver Disease*, 6th ed. Philadelphia: WB Saunders, 1998; with permission.

(< 300 IU/L) the AST:ALT ratio can be useful in differentiating various types of liver disease. AST is present in both the cytosol and the mitochondria, whereas ALT is present only in the mitochondria. Liver injury from alcohol primarily damages the mitochondria, so in alcoholic hepatitis, the AST:ALT ratio is usually > 2.0. In acute or chronic viral hepatitis, the ratio is reversed, with AST:ALT usually < 1. This ratio is less helpful in chronic liver disease because the AST:ALT ratio can be increased to > 1.0 in nonalcoholic cirrhosis.

If the elevation of AST or ALT is confirmed and drug-induced or alcoholic liver disease is suspected from the history, the offending agent(s) should be withdrawn, and tests repeated after 2 to 8 weeks. If the drug and alcohol history is negative, further evaluation of elevated aminotransferases should begin with testing for viral markers. Accurate serological tests for hepatitis A, B, and C are readily available.

Hepatitis C virus (HCV) infection affects an estimated 1.8% of the population and 14.4% of persons with ALT levels > 40 IU/L. It is the most common cause of chronic liver disease, cirrhosis, and liver transplantation in the United States. Given this high prevalence of HCV infection, serologic testing for HCV should be done early in the evaluation of a patient with chronically elevated aminotransferases. False-positive first generation anti-HCV antibody results have been described in patients with autoimmune chronic active hepatitis as well as other conditions associated with hyperglobulinemia.

In cases of suspected acute hepatitis, IgM antibody to hepatitis A virus should be performed to exclude hepatitis A. Hepatitis B surface antigen (HbsAg) and IgM antibody to hepatitis B core antigen (IgM anti-HBc) testing is done to evaluate acute hepatitis B. In chronic hepatitis B infection, HbsAg and anti-HBc antibody (total) are positive, whereas IgM anti-HBc antibody is usually undetectable. Acute hepatitis C can be present in the absence of antibody to the c100 antigen of the hepatitis C virus (anti-HCV antibody), but serial testing will usually confirm the diagnosis. It is also worth checking a Monospot, because acute Epstein-Barr virus infection can also elevate the aminotransferases.

Intravenous drug abusers and hemophiliacs with hepatitis B should also be evaluated for hepatitis D (Delta) virus infection. Hepatitis D (HDV) is an incomplete RNA virus that requires the presence of HbsAg to complete its replication and infect new liver cells. Co-infection or superinfection with HDV should be suspected in high-risk HbsAg-positive individuals and tested for by measuring anti-HDV antibody.

Further workup should be guided by the physician's findings from the history and physical examination (Fig. 5.1). Common causes of elevated aminotransferases are listed in Table 5.9.

Evaluation for Elevated Alkaline Phosphatase

An isolated elevated ALP level should always be rechecked, and hepatic origin suspected in patients who also have an elevation of GGT or 5'-NT (Fig. 5.2). It should be noted that mild elevations of ALP (< 1.5–2.0 times normal) are commonly found in routinely screened asymptomatic populations, and do not require further workup unless alcohol abuse is likely, or other laboratory tests are abnormal. An elevated ALP may be a physiologic finding in puberty or pregnancy, because ALP production tends to increase in tissues undergoing metabolic stimulation (see *Pathophysiology*). An increased ALP (with GGT) without alteration of other liver function tests may provide a useful clue to presence of hepatic infiltration, focal (e.g., metastatic) lesions, or early biliary cirrhosis.

Imaging studies should be considered early in the workup because of the high association between ALP elevations and biliary duct disease from inflammation, infiltrative processes (e.g., cancer or tuberculosis), or biliary obstruction from stones or tumors. Marked elevations of ALP are associated with extra- and intrahepatic cholesta-

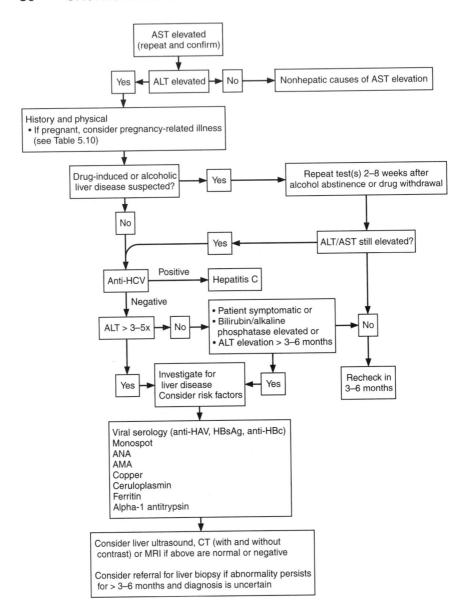

FIGURE 5.1. Approach to patient with elevated aspartate aminotransferase (AST). ALT, alanine aminotransferase; AMA, antimitochondrial antibody; ANA, antinuclear antibody; anti-HAV, hepatitis A antibody; CT, computed tomography; HbsAg, hepatitis B surface antigen; anti-HBc, hepatitis B core antibody; anti-HCV, hepatitis C antibody; MRI, magnetic resonance imaging. Adapted from Kamath PS. Clinical approach to the patient with abnormal liver test results. *Mayo Clin Proc,* 1996;71:1089–1095.

T ABLE 5.9. Possible causes of elevated aminotransferases

A	Autoimmune
B	Hepatitis B
C	Hepatitis C
D	Drugs or toxins
E	Ethanol
F	Fatty liver
G	Growths (tumors)
H	Hemodynamic (congestive heart failure)
I	Iron, copper, α-1 antitrypsin deficiency

From Quinn PG, Johnston DE. Detection of chronic liver disease: costs and benefits. *Gastroenterologist*, 1997; 5:58–77; with permission.

sis, diffuse infiltrating disease, and, occasionally, alcoholic hepatitis. Nonhepatic causes include Paget's disease and bony metastases.

Evaluation for Elevated Gamma Glutamyltransferase

Gamma glutamyltransferase is a membrane enzyme whose rise usually parallels the elevation of ALP. Although very sensitive to biliary tract disease, it is nonspecific. It can be elevated by a number of nonhepatic conditions (see *Pathophysiology*). In one study of patients with alcoholic liver disease, GGT was elevated in 52% of patients without known liver disease. It can be used to monitor abstinence from alcohol. Because of its lack of specificity, however, an extensive evaluation of isolated GGT elevations in otherwise healthy individuals is not warranted.

Imaging Studies

The role of hepatic imaging for mildly elevated concentrations of AST and ALT is less important than in cases of elevated ALP levels because of the higher association of the latter with cholestasis. Ultrasonography is generally a good first imaging test because it is useful to exclude focal liver disease (e.g., neoplasm or cyst), cholelithiasis, and biliary obstruction, and it is relatively inexpensive and noninvasive. However, a normal finding on ultrasound examination does not exclude the presence of diffuse or severe liver disease.

A suspected mass or biliary obstruction can be worked up using ultrasound, computed tomography (CT), magnetic resonance imaging (MRI), or endoscopic retrograde cholangiopancreatography (ERCP). Ultrasound, CT, and MRI can identify masses greater than 1 cm and can identify the cause of cholestasis in approximately 90% of cases. Ultrasound results are abnormal in about 65% of patients with chronically elevated liver function tests. An abnormal hyperechoic pattern will be found in 82% of patients who have a liver fat content above 10%. Approximately half of all patients with cirrhosis and 57% of patients with chronic liver inflammation have abnormal findings on ultrasound.

Abdominal CT or MRI can be helpful in the evaluation of patients with uncertain ultrasound findings. CT and MRI liver scans give comparable results; however, MRI is more expensive and cannot be used in patients with cardiac pacemakers and internal magnetic material (e.g., foreign bodies, clips). However, new advances in MRI technology (e.g., ultra-fast MRI) may lead to it eventually replacing CT for liver evaluation. ERCP identifies biliary duct strictures, cancer, and stones, but has a mortality rate of 0.1% to 0.2% and a morbidity rate of 2% to 3% (acute pancreatitis and cholangitis are the most frequent complications). Of attempted ERCPs, 10% to 20% are unsuccessful;

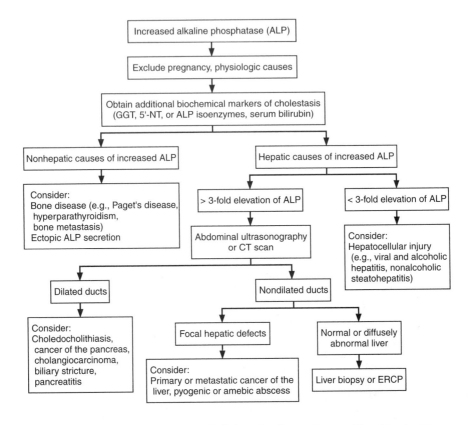

FIGURE 5.2. Evaluation for elevated alkaline phosphatase. Reprinted from Moseley RH. Approach to the patient with abnormal liver chemistries. In: Yamada T, ed. *Textbook of gastroenterology*, 3rd Ed. Philadelphia: Lippincott Williams & Wilkins, 1999:959.

if the ERCP fails, the patient may require percutaneous transhepatic cholangiography to achieve imaging. A new technique, magnetic resonance cholangiopancreatography, which is noninvasive and can be performed without using contrast material, is being increasingly used for biliary tract imaging.

Other imaging studies may add information to the workup. For example, finding emphysema on a chest x-ray film of a young individual with signs of cirrhosis supports the diagnosis of α_1-antitrypsin deficiency.

Liver Biopsy

The role of liver biopsy is either to document and stage the severity of a disease that abnormal test results identify (e.g., chronic hepatitis B or hepatitis C, hemochromatosis, or Wilson's disease) or to diagnose an underlying disease when the cause remains uncertain. In acute viral hepatitis, the liver enzymes can be elevated for more than 6 months. After this time, patients are considered to have chronic viral hepatitis and a liver biopsy is needed to distinguish chronic persistent hepatitis from chronic active hepatitis. It is an important diagnostic tool in the evaluation of persistent aminotransferase abnormalities. However, the morbidity and mortality of a liver biopsy is approximately 0.1%.

RISK FACTORS

General

Age and Gender

Wilson's disease typically presents during the second to fourth decades of life and almost never occurs beyond age 40. Hemochromatosis usually afflicts men in their 40s and 50s, whereas autoimmune hepatitis involves young or postmenopausal women. Nonalcoholic steatohepatitis (NASH) generally occurs in middle-aged obese women. Viral hepatitis A is primarily a disease of children and adolescents, but can infect anyone without previous immunity.

Medications and Alcohol

More than 300 different drugs have been associated with jaundice and abnormal liver function tests. The main classes of hepatotoxic drugs are phenothiazines, nonsteroidal antiinflammatory medications, tricyclic antidepressants, monoamine oxidase inhibitors, and antimicrobials. See Table 5.4 for a list of hepatotoxic drugs.

Alcoholic liver disease is suggested by a history of excessive alcohol ingestion (> 80–120 g/d) and is typically associated with modest increases in AST with normal or minimally elevated ALT (increased AST:ALT ratio). A frequently overlooked cause of markedly elevated aminotransferases in alcoholic patients is concomitant use of acetaminophen, even in therapeutic dosages.

Pregnancy

Pregnant patients are at risk for several liver diseases that are unique to pregnancy (Table 5.10).

1. Cholestasis of pregnancy (intrahepatic cholestasis of pregnancy, benign recurrent cholestasis)
   - Cholestasis of pregnancy is more common in Scandinavian countries, Bolivia, and Chile. It is also more common in twin pregnancies. It can be aggravated by progesterone therapy, which should probably be avoided in patients with a prior history of cholestasis of pregnancy.
   - It is characterized by the onset of severe pruritus in the third trimester of pregnancy. Itching is intense, especially at night and on the palms and soles. Cholestasis may be intense, and is associated with steatorrhea. Alkaline phosphatase and the aminotransferases are elevated, the latter occasionally ≥ 1,000 IU/L. GGT levels are usually normal or mildly elevated. Bilirubin is also elevated, but most patients are not jaundiced.
2. Acute fatty liver of pregnancy (AFLP)
   - Acute fatty liver of pregnancy (AFLP) is a rare form of acute hepatic failure, usually occurring in the third trimester. The incidence is approximately 1 of 13,000 deliveries. Maternal mortality rates range from 8% to 18%.
   - Primigravidas and patients with multiple gestations are at increased risk. It is more common with male fetuses.
3. Liver disease of preeclampsia or HELLP syndrome
   - Preeclampsia or eclampsia occurs in 5% to 7% of all pregnancies, usually in the third trimester. It is characterized by hypertension (blood pressure > 140/90) and proteinuria of ≥ 300 mg excreted in 24 hours. The liver is one of the target organs of preeclampsia, and elevations of aminotransferases are common. Rarely, severe liver involvement may lead to hepatic rupture. Risk factors for preeclampsia are nulliparity, plural gestation, maternal age less than 20 years or greater than 45 years, and a family history of preeclampsia. It is also associated with diabetes mellitus, hypertension, fetal hydrops, hydatidiform mole, polyhydramnios, and inadequate prenatal care.

T ABLE 5.10. Liver function abnormalities associated with pregnancy

Disease	Clinical features	Studies	Differential diagnosis / comments	Treatment
Hyperemesis gravidarum	Onset: first trimester Nausea and vomiting Mild jaundice	↑ AST (mild) ↑ Bilirubin (mild)	Differential diagnosis: viral hepatitis (mild) Normal liver biopsy	None or rehydration
Cholestasis of pregnancy (intrahepatic cholestasis of pregnancy, benign recurrent cholestasis)	Onset: third trimester More common in twin pregnancies Pruritus (may be severe) Jaundice (in ~10% of patients) Steatorrhea Liver/spleen not palpable No abdominal pain UTI may be associated with illness and can worsen severity	↑ ALP ↑ AST (mild, but occasionally to 1,000 IU/L or higher); ↑ ALT (>10 times normal in 40% of cases) GGT normal or modestly elevated Bilirubin elevated (<5 mg/dl)	Differential diagnosis: pruritus gravidarum, viral hepatitis, biliary obstruction (e.g., cholelithiasis), primary biliary cirrhosis, benign recurrent intrahepatic cholestasis. (Note: Pregnancy can exacerbate underlying subclinical cholestatic illness) May recur with subsequent pregnancies or with use of OCP; 60% to 70% of patients affected in their initial pregnancies have a recurrence Rapid remission after delivery May be an increase in fetal distress, prematurity, and unexplained stillbirth	Symptomatic medications: Hydroxyzine (Atarax, Vistaril) for pruritus Ursodeoxycholic acid (URSO) Cholestyramine (Questran) Barbiturates Close fetal monitoring No need to immediately induce pregnancy; some recommend elective planned delivery after achieving fetal lung maturity Check for UTI

| HELLP syndrome (usually associated with severe preeclampsia) | Onset: third trimester (usually after 27th week); approximately two-thirds of cases present antepartum, one-third postpartum
Occurs in almost 20% of women with severe preeclampsia
Epigastric, RUQ abdominal or epigastric (65%)
Nausea or vomiting (36%)
Headache (31%)
Bleeding (9%)
Jaundice (5%)[a]
Malaise, blurred vision, thirst | ↑ AST (median 250 IU/L; range 70–6,000 IU/L)
↑ Bilirubin (median 1.5 mg/dl; range 0.5–25 mg/dl)
↓ Platelets (median 50,000; range 7,000–99,000)[a]
Hemolysis (fragmented cells on blood smear)
↑ LDH | Differential diagnosis: idiopathic thrombocytopenic purpura, thrombotic thrombocytopenic purpura, antiphospholipid antibody syndrome, acute fatty liver of pregnancy
Liver disease ranges from mild to extremely severe
Complications:
DIC (21%)
Abruptio placentae (16%)
Acute renal failure (8%)
Rare complications:
Subcapsular hematoma of liver with or without hepatic rupture (1%); necrotic liver infarction
Mortality (1%)[a] | Intensive care support
Some patients may require platelet transfusion or dialysis
Corticosteroids improve laboratory abnormalities and may speed fetal lung maturity
Early delivery is recommended in severe cases with maternal or fetal distress; milder cases may be observed without delivery |

continued

T ABLE 5.10 continued. **Liver function abnormalities associated with pregnancy**

Disease	Clinical features	Studies	Differential diagnosis/comments	Treatment
Acute fatty liver of pregnancy (AFLP)	Onset: third trimester (usually 34th to 37th weeks, rarely as early as 19th week) Jaundice Pruritus Nausea and vomiting Abdominal pain Acute hepatic failure Bleeding diathesis Confusion, coma	↑ AST (300–500 IU/L) ↑ ALP (2–3 normal) ↑ Bilirubin (3–25 mg/dl) ↑ Protime ↓ Fibrinogen ↑ BUN, creatinine, uric acid Liver biopsy characterized by microvesicular fatty infiltration prominent in central zone	Differential diagnosis: viral hepatitis (check serologies, consider hepatitis E and herpes simplex hepatitis, which can be very severe during pregnancy), drug-induced liver injury, HELLP syndrome Early delivery advocated; fetal mortality 18% to 23%, maternal mortality 8% to 18%, maternal survival nears 100% with prompt diagnosis and care Often associated with preeclampsia No recurrence with future pregnancies One study showed prevalence in 1 of 6,692 deliveries	Early delivery Intensive care support
Tetracycline-induced	Onset: usually third trimester Presentation similar to acute fatty liver of pregnancy	Similar to acute fatty liver of pregnancy	Histology identical to acute fatty liver Usually seen with TCN doses >3 g daily, either orally or intravenously	Cessation of tetracycline (tetracycline should *never* be given to pregnant women)

AST, aspartate aminotransferase; ALP, alkaline phosphatase; BUN, blood urea nitrogen; DIC, disseminated intravascular coagulation; GGT, gamma glutamyl transpepidase; HELLP, hemolysis, elevated liver enzymes, low platelets; LDH, lactate dehydrogenase; OCP, oral contraceptive pills; RUQ, right upper quadrant; TCN, tetracycline; UTI, urinary tract infection.

[a]Data on HELLP syndrome from Sibai BH, Ramadan MK, Usta I, et al. Maternal morbidity and mortality in 442 pregnancies with hemolysis, elevated liver enzymes, and low platelets (HELLP syndrome). Am J Obstet Gynecol 1993;169:100–106.

Table adapted from Anderson PB. Liver dysfunction. In: Reilly BM, ed. Practical strategies in outpatient medicine, 2nd ed. Philadelphia: WB Saunders, 1991.

- HELLP syndrome occurs in approximately 0.2% to 0.6% of all pregnancies, and occurs in 4% to 12% of women with preeclampsia or eclampsia. However, it may also be associated with AFLP, or may occur alone.
- Risk factors for HELLP syndrome include multiparity, maternal age > 25 years, white race, and a history of poor pregnancy outcome.

Specific Diseases

Viral Hepatitis A, B, and C

Risk factors for hepatitis A, B, and C are listed in Table 5.11. All of these viruses can be passed between sex partners; however, whereas hepatitis A is primarily transmitted through the fecal-oral route, hepatitis B (HBV) and hepatitis C (HCV) are primarily transmitted through blood and body secretions. HBV is much more highly transmissible through sexual contact than HCV. The available data indicate that transmission does occur sexually from patients with HCV, although with a very low frequency. In the United States, 10% to 15% of persons reported to have acute hepatitis C have reported a history of high-risk sexual behaviors that include contracting a sexually transmitted disease and having unprotected sex with multiple partners in the absence of percutaneous risk factors. Two thirds of these persons had an anti-HCV–positive partner.

Previously hospitalized patients are at increased risk for viral hepatitis. In one study of medical outpatients with elevated ALT, evidence of acute or chronic hepatitis B infection could be detected serologically in 6%; if ALT was more than fivefold elevated, hepatitis B could be detected in 15%.

Fatty Liver (Hepatic Steatosis) and Nonalcoholic Steatohepatitis

Fatty liver, or hepatic steatosis, is perhaps the most common cause of mildly elevated liver enzymes in the United States. It is characterized by fatty infiltration of the liver. Nonalcoholic steatohepatitis (NASH) is similar to fatty liver, but has a more aggressive course and can progress to cirrhosis in up to 20% of patients. The mechanism is not well understood. In populations at risk, such as patients with type 2 diabetes mellitus, prevalence of NASH can be as high as 50%. Risk factors for both disorders include diabetes, hyperlipidemia, jejunoileal bypass surgery, corticosteroid therapy, alcohol abuse, starvation, obesity, and vitamin A toxicity.

Hemochromatosis

Hemochromatosis is a slowly progressive genetic disease characterized by abnormalities of iron storage. It is inherited in an autosomal recessive pattern, with a gene frequency of approximately 6% and a disease prevalence (homozygous state) of between 3 and 5 cases per 1,000 persons. Northern European ancestry is the primary risk factor. In men, onset of disease is usually in the third and fourth decades of life, whereas menses generally protects women until menopause. The disease is often asymptomatic until a significant amount of iron has accumulated in the tissues, usually by age 40 to 60 years.

Alcoholic Liver Disease

Alcoholic liver disease is suggested by a history of excessive alcohol consumption, but occasionally this history is lacking. It can range from simple fatty liver to alcoholic hepatitis; cirrhosis develops in only 20% to 30% of patients who consume a substantial amount of alcohol, defined as more than a decade of 60 to 80 g/d alcohol in men, and 20 to 40 g/d in women. A standard drink contains 12 g alcohol; this equals one 12-oz beer, 5-oz glass of wine, or 1.5 oz distilled spirits. Other risk factors include female gender, chronic viral hepatitis (especially HCV), hemochromatosis, and certain medications (e.g., methotrexate) that potentiate the harmful effects of alcohol.

T ABLE 5.11. At-risk groups

HEPATITIS A
Household/sexual contacts of infected persons
Ingestion of uncooked shellfish (e.g., clams, mussels, oysters)
Living or traveling in places with poor sanitation or overcrowding
Persons living in American Indian reservations, Alaskan Native villages, and other regions with endemic
    hepatitis A
Primate handlers
During outbreaks: day care center employees or attendees, homosexually active men, injecting drug users

HEPATITIS B
Injection drug users
Sexually active heterosexuals
Homosexually active men
Infants/children of immigrants from disease-endemic areas (i.e., Africa, China, Middle East, South America,
    Southeast Asia, or the Pacific Islands)
Low socioeconomic level
Sexual/household contacts of infected persons
Infants born to infected mothers
Healthcare workers
Hemodialysis Patients

HEPATITIS C
Injecting drug users
Hemodialysis patients
Healthcare workers
Sexual contacts of infected persons
Household exposure (sharing razor or toothbrush with a hepatitis C virus-infected person)
Persons with multiple sex partners
Recipients of transfusions or organ donation before July 1992
Recipients of clotting factors made before 1987
Infants born to infected mothers
Tattooing or body piercing in unsanitary conditions
Intranasal cocaine users

Autoimmune Hepatitis
Typically a disease of young women, although individuals of both sexes and older ages may be affected by autoimmune hepatitis.

α_1-*Antitrypsin Deficiency*
Alpha$_1$ antitrypsin deficiency is a genetic disease; a family history of α_1-antitrypsin deficiency is a risk factor.

Primary Biliary Cirrhosis
Primary biliary cirrhosis is a disease of middle-aged women characterized by cholestasis and an elevated ALP level. It is often found in patients with autoimmune disorders

TABLE 5.12. Differential diagnosis and evaluation of patients with chronically elevated liver enzymes (>3–6 months) after discontinuation of all hepatotoxic drugs

Disease	Clinical features	Laboratory evaluation	Differential diagnosis / comments	Treatment
Alcoholic liver disease	History of ethanol ingestion (>80–120 g/dl) Jaundice, fever, RUQ abdominal pain Hepatomegaly Cirrhosis, ascites Portal hypertension	High GGT High MCV AST:ALT ratio >2:1	Differential diagnosis: may be difficult to distinguish from NASH or hemochromatosis. Liver biopsy may be helpful.	Prednisone in selected cases of severe alcoholic hepatitis Discontinue alcohol use
Fatty liver NASH	Female gender (more common in women) Obesity Diabetes	Mild GGT, AST, and ALT elevation Glucose intolerance Liver biopsy shows fatty infiltration	Differential diagnosis: may be difficult to distinguish from alcoholic hepatitis	Control of underlying obesity or diabetes
Autoimmune hepatitis	Female gender (more common in women) Fatigue, amenorrhea May have associated thyroiditis, arthritis, vasculitis, Sjögren's syndrome	+ ANA (80%) + SMA (70%) High gamma globulin levels (>3 g/dl)	Differential diagnosis: Primary biliary cirrhosis Primary sclerosing cholangitis Chronic viral hepatitis Autoimmune cholangitis	Prednisone alone or in combination with azathioprine (Imuran) is effective: overall 10-year survival is ~93%
Primary biliary cirrhosis	Female gender (>90% in women) Fatigue, pruritus May have associated thyroiditis, arthritis, Sjögren's syndrome, scleroderma, renal tubular acidosis	High ALP (often >800 IU/L) + AMA (>90%) High IgG levels + ANA (33%) Must rule out extrahepatic biliary obstruction	Differential diagnosis: Extrahepatic biliary obstruction Primary sclerosing cholangitis Drug-induced cholestasis Autoimmune hepatitis Granulomatous hepatitis Chronic hepatitis B or C Alcoholic hepatitis Sarcoidosis	Ursodeoxycholic acid (URSO) appears to be the most beneficial. Controversial: Corticosteroids Colchicine Methotrexate Liver transplantation is treatment of choice for advanced disease.

continued

T ABLE 5.12 continued. Differential diagnosis and evaluation of patients with chronically elevated liver enzymes (>3–6 months) after discontinuation of all hepatotoxic drugs

Disease	Clinical features	Laboratory evaluation	Differential diagnosis/comments	Treatment
Primary sclerosing cholangitis	Young male Often associated with inflammatory bowel disease, especially ulcerative colitis Fatigue, pruritus, jaundice Onset insidious	High ALP Mild elevations of AST and ALT AMA Liver biopsy and ERCP help confirm diagnosis	Differential diagnosis: Primary biliary cirrhosis Wilson's disease	Ursodeoxycholic acid (URSO) Cholestyramine (Questran) Biliary strictures managed with endoscopic balloon dilation/stent Liver transplantation
Chronic hepatitis B	Nonspecific symptoms of malaise, anorexia, and fatigue Post-transfusion IV drug abuse, unsafe sex practices	Moderate AST elevation HBsAg+ Anti-HBcAb+	Increased risk of hepatocellular carcinoma HBV infection may occur in up to one-third of patients with HCV infection	Prednisone of no benefit Interferon alfa-2b (Intron A) Lamivudine (Epivir)
Chronic hepatitis C	Nonspecific symptoms of malaise, anorexia, and fatigue Post-transfusion IV drug abuse	Moderate AST elevation Anti-HCV+	Up to 70% of patients are asymptomatic Increased risk of hepatocellular carcinoma HCV infection accounts for 25% of adults referred for liver transplant in the United States	Interferon alfa-2a (Roferon-A) Interferon alfa-2b Interferon alfacon-1 (Infergen) Interferon alfa-2b plus ribavirin (Rebetron)

Disease	Clinical features	Laboratory evaluation	Comments	Treatment
Hemochromatosis	Positive family history Systemic illness (heart, pancreas) Arthritis	Iron/TIBC >0.6 Ferritin >200 µg/dl in men; >150 µg/dl in women C2824/H630 genotyping	Liver biopsy diagnostic: elevated hepatic iron index (iron concentration: age) Family members should be screened Increased risk of hepatocellular carcinoma	Phlebotomy Deferoxamine [(Desferal); iron-chelating drug] for cardiac disease
Wilson's disease	Young patients Kayser-Fleischer rings Neuropsychiatric symptoms	Serum ceruloplasmin <20 µg/dl Low serum copper Hepatic copper elevated (liver biopsy)		Penicillamine (Cuprimine) Trientine (Syprine) Zinc acetate (Galzin)
α_1-antitrypsin deficiency	Positive family history of liver and lung disease Hepatosplenomegaly, portal hypertension Jaundice, poor weight gain in children	Serum protein electrophoresis Serum α_1-antitrypsin level Pheno typing	Differential diagnosis: Chronic viral hepatitis	Genetic counseling Liver transplantation

ALP, alkaline phosphatase; ALT, alanine transaminase (SGPT); AMA, antimitochondrial antibody; ANA, antinuclear antibody; anti-HCV, hepatitis C virus antibody; AST, aspartate aminotransferase (SGOT); ERCP, endoscopic retrograde cholangiopancreatography; GGT, gamma glutamyl-transferase; HBcAb, hepatitis B core antibody; HbsAg, hepatitis B surface antigen; HBV, hepatitis B virus; HCV, hepatitis C virus; IgG, gamma G immunoglobulin; IV, intravenous; MCV, mean corpuscular volume; NASH, nonalcoholic steatohepatitis; RUQ, right upper quadrant; SMA, smooth muscle antibody; TIBC, total iron-binding capacity.

Adapted from Anderson PB. Liver dysfunction. In Reilly BM, ed. *Practical Strategies in Outpatient Medicine*, 2nd ed. Philadelphia: WB Saunders; 1991.

such as scleroderma, CREST syndrome (calcinosis cutis, Raynaud's phenomenon, esophageal dysmotility, sclerodactyly, telangiectasia), Sjögren's syndrome, and autoimmune thyroiditis.

Primary Sclerosing Cholangitis

Primary sclerosing cholangitis often occurs in association with inflammatory bowel disease, especially ulcerative colitis, or with multifocal fibrosclerosis syndromes such as retroperitoneal, mediastinal, or periureteral fibrosis, Riedel's struma, or pseudotumor of the orbit. Primary sclerosing cholangitis is often a complication of acquired immunodeficiency syndrome (AIDS); often these patients have infections with cytomegalovirus or cryptosporidia, which may indicate an association with these infections.

Wilson's Disease

Wilson's disease is a rare inherited metabolic disorder of copper metabolism in children and young adults, and should be considered in patients under age 40 years with unexplained abnormalities of aminotransferases or signs of hepatic injury. The only risk factor is a positive family history of the disorder.

DIFFERENTIAL DIAGNOSIS

Table 5.12 lists the differential diagnosis and evaluation of patients with chronically elevated liver enzyme tests that persist for more than 3 to 6 months. Specific diseases are discussed in more detail below.

Viral Hepatitis A, B, and C

Findings of serologic tests will usually distinguish the various types of viral hepatitis, and the tests should be performed early in the workup of patients with elevated liver enzymes. False-positive anti-HCV tests have been reported in patients who have autoimmune hepatitis. Findings that support a true-positive result include persistence of anti-HCV on serial testing, confirmation of reactivity by neutralizing or immunoblot assays, and the presence of HCV RNA by the polymerase chain reaction.

Between 0.2% and 0.9% of the general population have positive reactions to HBV surface antigen. Acute hepatitis B progresses to chronic infection (usually defined by elevated aminotransferase levels for more than 6 months) in 5% of infected adults and 80% to 90% of infected infants. Of chronic hepatitis B infections, 10% advance to cirrhosis. Hepatitis C, by contrast, progresses to chronic hepatitis in at least 50% of cases of acute HCV infection.

Fatty Liver (Hepatic Steatosis) and Nonalcoholic Steatohepatitis (NASH)

Nonalcoholic steatohepatitis and steatonecrosis are terms recently coined to describe a form of fatty liver disease with a potentially progressive course. Their mechanism is not well understood: theories include abnormalities of lipid metabolism with increased hepatic lipid peroxidation, activated fibrocytes, and abnormal patterns of cytokine production. Data from a few limited natural history studies suggest that simple steatosis has a benign course, whereas nonalcoholic steatohepatitis or steatonecrosis can progress to cirrhosis in 10% to 20% of patients. The diagnosis of NASH can only be established in patients who do not consume significant amounts of alcohol.

Liver biopsy findings are nearly identical to those associated with alcoholic hepatitis, but the natural history is much more benign. NASH, also called fatty hepatitis or fatty cirrhosis when regenerative nodules are present, is associated with significant damage to the liver but can be difficult to distinguish clinically or biochemically from simple fatty liver. Laboratory profiles typically show less than three times elevation of AST or ALT, mild elevation of ALP, and normal serum bilirubin and serum albumin. Viral serological testing is essential to distinguish fatty liver and NASH from chronic viral hepatitis.

Hemochromatosis

Three tests should be done to evaluate for hemochromatosis: serum iron, transferrin saturation (serum iron and total iron-binding capacity), and ferritin. The diagnosis of homochromatosis should be suggested if the serum iron is more than 175 µg/dl, the transferrin saturation is more than 60%, or the ferritin is more than 200 µg/L in men or more than 150 µg/L in women. The combination of an elevated transferrin saturation and an elevated ferritin level in an apparently healthy individual is 93% sensitive for hereditary hemochromatosis. Genotyping for C2824 and H63D can now be used to confirm the diagnosis of hemochromatosis. Patients with elevated iron studies can be diagnosed if they are homozygous for C2824 or C2824/H63D heterzygous. Accurate diagnosis with other genotypes requires biopsy and measuring the hepatic iron index.

Patients who develop cirrhosis from hemochromatosis are at risk for liver failure and hepatocellular carcinoma. In untreated patients, the most common causes of death are heart failure (30%), hepatocellular carcinoma (30%), and portal hypertension (25%). Elevated iron stores increase the risk for arthritis because of iron deposits in joints and for sexual dysfunction because of iron loading in the pituitary. All first-degree relatives should be screened with a liver panel, serum iron, total iron-binding capacity, and ferritin.

Alcoholic Liver Disease

Alcoholic liver disease is typically associated with a modestly increased AST with a normal or minimally elevated ALT (increased AST:ALT ratio). An AST:ALT ratio of more than 2:1 is suggestive of alcoholic liver disease. In one study, 70% of patients with alcoholic liver disease had a ratio greater than 2, compared with only 8% of patients with chronic active hepatitis, 4% with viral hepatitis, and none with obstructive jaundice. It should be noted that even in the presence of a characteristic AST:ALT pattern, up to 17% of alcoholic patients may have other (nonalcoholic) liver diseases after liver biopsy is performed.

It can be difficult to distinguish alcoholic liver disease from NASH or hemochromatosis; liver biopsy can often be helpful, although it cannot reliably distinguish alcoholic liver disease from NASH.

Autoimmune Hepatitis

Autoimmune hepatitis is a rare autoimmune disease. It may be associated with hyperglobulinemia, splenomegaly, and other autoimmune features (arthritis, rash, thyroiditis, Coomb's positive hemolytic anemia), but may manifest only as chronic liver disease. Although typically a disease of young women, individuals of both sexes and older ages can be affected. The diagnosis relies on the presence of autoantibodies in the serum. Homogeneous antinuclear antibody (ANA) is found in 80% of those affected; 70% have titers of smooth muscle antibody, and 80% have hypergammaglobulinemia. Antismooth muscle antibody (ASMA), or liver-kidney-microsomal antibody (LKM) in association with characteristic liver biopsy findings (portal and periportal inflammation with lymphocytes and plasma cells and piecemeal necrosis of heptocytes) confirms the diagnosis.

The differential diagnosis of autoimmune hepatitis includes primary biliary cirrhosis, primary sclerosing cholangitis, chronic viral hepatitis, and autoimmune cholangitis.

α_1-Antitrypsin Deficiency

α_1-Antitrypsin deficiency affects only 1% of all adults and children with chronic liver disease. The family history may be positive for chronic lung disease. Although it can mimic chronic viral hepatitis, a diminished α_1-globulin fraction is often present on serum protein electrophoresis and may be confirmed with an α_1-antitrypsin level and phenotyping. In young, nonsmoking patients with evidence of emphysema on a chest x-ray film, the possibility of α_1- antitrypsin deficiency should be considered. Furthermore, the disease should be considered in any patient presenting with hepatosplenomegaly, cirrhosis, portal hypertension, or chronic hepatitis with negative serological tests. Children may present with jaundice and poor weight gain.

Primary Biliary Cirrhosis

The differential diagnosis of primary biliary cirrhosis includes other causes of chronic cholestatic disease, such as extrahepatic biliary obstruction, primary sclerosing cholangitis, drug-induced cholestasis, autoimmune hepatitis, granulomatous hepatitis, sarcoidosis, chronic viral hepatitis, and alcoholic hepatitis. Diagnosis can be difficult because of overlap with other syndromes, especially primary sclerosing cholangitis. An elevated serum IgG antimitochondrial antibody titer (positive in 85% to 95% of cases) is a characteristic finding in primary biliary cirrhosis that is rarely found in other forms of liver disease. Liver biopsy shows periductal granulomas and lymph follicles adjacent to affected bile ducts—findings also seen in graft-versus-host disease, suggesting an immune defect. Imaging studies and cholangiography help distinguish primary biliary cirrhosis from primary sclerosing cholangitis.

Primary Sclerosing Cholangitis

Primary sclerosing cholangitis is disease of young men with ulcerative colitis. It is characterized by progressive sclerosing, inflammation, and obliteration of the extrahepatic duct and often the intrahepatic bile duct. It often presents with symptoms of biliary obstruction and an elevated ALP and bilirubin level. It is slowly progressive, with a mean period of 4 to 10 years from diagnosis to time of death. Patients invariably require liver transplantation. It can be confused with primary biliary cirrhosis and Wilson's disease, because hepatic copper can be elevated in both primary sclerosing cholangitis and primary biliary cirrhosis. However, serum copper and ceruloplasmin levels are usually increased, unlike either Wilson's disease or primary biliary cirrhosis, and the mitochondrial antibody test is negative. ERCP is required for diagnosis, which shows thickened ducts with narrow, beaded lumina.

Wilson's Disease

Wilson's disease, a rare inherited metabolic disorder of copper metabolism in children and young adults, is usually slowly progressive and can have neurologic, psychiatric, hepatic, or renal manifestations.

Serum copper is reduced, and 24-hour urinary copper increased. Serum ceruloplasmin is typically reduced, but can be in the low-normal range in patients with active liver disease. In 90% to 95% of patients with Wilson's disease, the ceruloplasmin level is less than 20 mg/dl, and 5% to 10% have low-normal levels (21–30 mg/dl). Other laboratory findings are hypouricemia and hemolytic anemia. Liver biopsy, which reveals elevated hepatic copper levels, confirms the diagnosis.

Drugs

Many illnesses can resemble drug-induced hepatitis. Often, the diagnosis requires a period of observation during which the liver abnormalities resolve after removal of a possibly hepatotoxic drug, along with normal findings on viral serologies and other liver tests.

Pregnancy-Related Conditions

Cholestasis of pregnancy can resemble primary biliary cirrhosis, benign recurrent intrahepatic cholestasis, viral hepatitis, and biliary obstruction. Underlying cholestatic illnesses (e.g., primary biliary cirrhosis) can be exacerbated by pregnancy.

Acute fatty liver of pregnancy (AFLP) can be confused with viral hepatitis (check serologies: consider hepatitis E and herpes simplex hepatitis, which can be very severe in pregnancy), drug-induced liver injury, and HELLP syndrome. The patient's history, physical examination, and laboratory profile findings will usually rule out viral causes of liver failure. Differentiation from severe HELLP syndrome may be particularly difficult, because AFLP patients may develop disseminated intravascular coagulation (DIC) with thrombocytopenia. Liver biopsy is helpful, but often dangerous, and the diagnosis often must rest on clinical grounds.

The differential diagnosis of liver disease of preeclampsia or HELLP syndrome includes idiopathic thrombocytopenic purpura, thrombotic thrombocytopenic purpura, and antiphospholipid antibody syndrome. AFLP is usually associated with more severe liver failure, without thrombocytopenia.

Other

Other causes of elevated liver enzymes are syphilis, tuberculosis, sarcoidosis, and neoplasm.

REFERRAL

The family physician, following the guidelines in the algorithms, can generally do the initial evaluation in patients who are not seriously ill. Often, if the patient is asymptomatic and the probable diagnosis is alcohol or drug use, viral hepatitis, or fatty liver, a period of observation of up to 6 months is reasonable. If, however, the patient is symptomatic and the liver enzymes remain elevated, or with strong suspicion of a disease that requires treatment, further evaluation will be needed, possibly including liver biopsy. If the diagnosis remains elusive after preliminary testing and observation and the liver enzymes remain elevated, consider referral to a gastroenterologist.

MANAGEMENT

Management of elevated liver enzymes depends on the specific diagnosis. An accurate diagnosis is important to establish prognosis and to identify illnesses for which beneficial treatments are available. Some treatment modalities are listed below.

Viral Hepatitis A

Supportive measures are the only treatment necessary in most cases of acute HAV infection. In patients with severe cholestasis, a short course of prednisolone (30 mg/d with a taper) may reduce the severity of symptoms (e.g., pruritus and malaise) and reduce the serum bilirubin level. Prolonged administration of corticosteroids is not recommended. Acute liver failure should prompt early consideration of liver transplantation.

For postexposure prophylaxis, gamma globulin (IG) is recommended (0.02 ml/kg intramuscular). Preexposure prophylaxis with hepatitis A vaccine is effective; two doses of vaccine are required, 6 to 12 months apart. Many authorities now recommend that patients who are positive for human immunodeficiency virus (HIV) or who are HBV- or HCV-positive should also receive hepatitis A vaccine, because superinfection with hepatitis A can create serious illness in patients with preexisting compromise of the liver or immune system.

Viral Hepatitis B

No treatment regimen has been shown to be of benefit for acute hepatitis B.

For chronic hepatitis B virus (HBV) infection, interferon alfa-2b (Intron A) has been shown to be beneficial in a number of studies. It is indicated for the treatment of chronic hepatitis B in patients aged 1 year or older with compensated liver disease. Patients who have been serum HBsAg-positive for at least 6 months and have evidence of HBV replication (serum HBeAg-positive) with elevated serum ALT are candidates for treatment. Studies in these patients demonstrated that interferon alfa-2b therapy can produce virologic remission of this disease (loss of serum HbeAg and HBV DNA) in 30% to 40% of patients and normalization of serum aminotransferases. Treatment resulted in the loss of serum HBsAg in 5% to 10% of responding patients.

The dosage of interferon alfa-2b is 5 million IU daily or 10 million IU three times a week, given subcutaneously or intramuscularly for 4 months. Serum ALT levels can rise dramatically during therapy, which may signal a response to therapy; however, such flares are not well tolerated by patients with cirrhosis.

Oral lamivudine (Epivir) inhibits HBV replication by interfering with DNA polymerase. It has fewer side effects than interferon alpha-2b and is easier to administer. It produces loss of serum HbeAg and HBV DNA in 16% to 32% of patients, and can be effective in patients who fail to respond to interferon alpha-2b. However, the optimal length of therapy is unknown. Mutant forms of HBV can appear during therapy, which may result in reappearance of HBV DNA. Because of relapses, long-term therapy with lamivudine may be necessary. The dosage is 100 mg/d by mouth. It is supplied as 100 mg tablets or 5 mg/ml oral solution.

Chronic Hepatitis C

Antiviral therapy in chronic HCV patients aims to normalize ALT values and produce loss of HCV RNA. Three interferon preparations have been approved for therapy: interferon alfa-2a (Roferon-A), interferon alfa-2b (Intron-A), and interferon alfacon-1 (Infergen).

The recommended regimen for interferon alfa-2a or interferon alfa-2b therapy is 3 million IU administered subcutaneously or intramuscularly three times a week for 12 months, which can be extended, depending on the response. Interferon alfacon-1 is given in a dose of 9 μg subcutaneously three times a week for an initial course of 24 weeks. If patients have persistently abnormal ALT levels and detectable serum HCV RNA after 3 months of interferon therapy, treatment should be discontinued. Approximately 50% of treated patients have an initial response, with normalization of serum ALT activity and a loss or decrease of serum HCV RNA at the end of therapy. After interferon therapy is discontinued, however, more than one half of patients who responded to treatment relapse, with recurrence of elevated ALT levels and reappearance of serum HCV RNA. Thus, only 15% to 25% of treated patients have a sustained response 1 or more years after therapy ends.

Ribavirin (Virazole), a nucleoside analog, has been evaluated in clinical trials alone and in combination with interferon. In studies of patients treated with ribavirin alone, results demonstrated a decrease in ALT activity in approximately one third of patients, but no change in viral replication. In addition, when treatment was withdrawn, all patients relapsed, with recurrence of elevated ALT levels. Thus, monotherapy with ribavirin is not useful in the treatment of chronic hepatitis C.

The results of studies of patients treated with a combination of oral ribavirin and subcutaneous interferon alfa-2b, however, demonstrated a substantial increase in sustained response rates compared with interferon therapy alone, reaching 40% to 50% of patients. As with interferon-alone therapy, however, combination therapy in patients with genotype 1 (the most common strain of HCV in the United States) is not as successful; sustained response rates among these patients are still less than 30%. Combination therapy with interferon alfa-2b and ribavirin (Rebetron) is now licensed for the treatment of chronic hepatitis C in patients who have compensated liver disease previously untreated with alpha interferon or who have relapsed following alpha interferon therapy.

The dosage for interferon alfa-2b is 3 million IU three times weekly subcutaneously, plus daily oral ribavirin dosed according to weight. Patients weighing ≤ 75 kg take two 200-mg capsules in the morning, and three 200-mg capsules in the evening; patients > 75 kg take three 200-mg capsules twice daily. Therapy is continued for 24 to 48 weeks.

Fatty Liver

Weight reduction, diabetes control, and treatment of hyperlipidemia have limited benefit, but should be undertaken. If patients can lose 10% or more of their body weight over a period of 6 to 12 months, ALT concentrations will return to normal when fatty liver is the only underlying hepatic condition.

Wilson's Disease

Three generally recognized substances are available to treat Wilson's disease: penicillamine (Cuprimine), trientine hydrochloride (Syprine), and zinc acetate (Galzin).

Penicillamine is the initial drug of choice; it works by increasing urinary excretion of copper. The dose is 1 to 2 g/d in four divided doses taken a half hour before meals and at bedtime. Pyridoxine (vitamin B6) is usually added in a dose of 25 mg daily because of the antipyridoxine effect of penicillamine.

Trientine hydrochloride chelates and mobilizes stored copper. It is less toxic than penicillamine, but is also less effective. The recommended initial dose of trientine is 500 to 750 mg daily for pediatric patients aged 12 years or under and 750 to 1,250 mg daily for adults given in divided doses two, three, or four times daily. This can be increased to a maximum of 2000 mg/d for adults or 1,500 mg/d for pediatric patients.

Zinc acetate prevents reaccumulation of copper by inhibiting copper absorption in the intestine. The usual dosage is 150 mg daily in three doses.

With effective treatment, most patients with Wilson's disease live normal, healthy lives, whereas untreated patients rarely survive their 30th year. Early treatment is critical; the outcome is best for patients whose disease is diagnosed and who begin treatment when they are presymptomatic. However, whether routine institution of chelator therapy in infancy is advantageous remains unknown. Likewise, the potential role for gene transfer therapy remains uncertain. Although drug treatment simply to interfere with absorption of dietary copper is now rarely used, most patients should eliminate copper-rich foods from their diet. These foods include organ meats, shellfish, nuts, chocolate, and mushrooms. Vegetarians require specific dietary counseling. If patients have reason to believe that their drinking water is high in copper, the water should be analyzed and a copper-removing device may be needed in the plumbing system.

Hemochromatosis

Prompt diagnosis with removal of excessive tissue iron by phlebotomy in the early stages of accumulation prevents permanent organ damage and manifestations of hemochromatosis. Weekly phlebotomy of 500 mL of blood is usually well tolerated and should be continued until ferritin levels are below 50 ng/mL, which may require up to 2 years of "induction" therapy. Maintenance therapy is continued for the life of the patient by phlebotomy of one or two units of blood three to four times a year to maintain the ferritin level below 50 ng/mL. Patients with advanced liver disease or hepatocellular carcinoma may require liver transplantation.

Autoimmune Hepatitis

Prednisone alone, or in combination with azathioprine (Imuran), is effective for autoimmune hepatitis and induces remission in 65% of patients within 3 years. The overall 10-year survival for treated patients is 93%.

Relapse occurs in 50% of patients within 6 months, but these patients usually respond to retreatment. Patients who relapse at least twice require chronic maintenance therapy with either prednisone or azathioprine.

Primary Biliary Cirrhosis

The course is chronic: the asymptomatic period can range from one to 20 years. Ursodeoxycholic acid (URSO) appears to be the most beneficial treatment, producing clinical and biochemical improvement. Corticosteroids have shown benefit in small studies, but further research is needed. Other therapies, such as colchicine, methotrexate, cyclosporine (Sandimmune), azothiaprine, and penicillamine (Cuprimine) are of questionable benefit and are not approved for treatment of this disorder. Many patients will eventually require liver transplant, which is the treatment of choice for advanced disease.

Primary Sclerosing Cholangitis

Primary sclerosing cholangitis is a progressive disease that usually results in liver failure and the need for liver transplantation. Although few treatment options are available, the diagnosis does enable patients to plan their life and allows the physician to consider experimental treatment [e.g., ursodeoxycholic acid (URSO)], and to anticipate and treat complications [e.g., treat pruritis with cholestyramine (Questran)]. Recurrent bacterial cholangitis is treated with antibiotics. Biliary duct carcinoma complicates approximately 10% of cases. A dominant common bile duct stricture resulting in jaundice or bacterial cholangitis can be managed with endoscopic balloon dilation, with or without stent placement. Patients invariably require liver transplantation: in one study, the mean time from diagnosis to liver transplantation was 5.8 years.

Alcoholic Liver Disease

The cornerstone of treatment is abstinence from alcohol, which can improve outcome regardless of the stage of illness. A variety of medications have been studied. Corticosteroids may be of some benefit in a sub-group of patients with the most severe liver disease, but they do not appear to be universally effective. Liver transplantation is an option for selected patients meeting rigorous criteria.

α_1–Antitrypsin Deficiency

Therapy for α_1-antitrypsin deficiency is directed at treatment of lung disease, including treatment of infections, smoking cessation counseling, and treatment of airway obstruction. The only effective therapy for end-stage liver disease is liver transplantation. Gene transfer therapy to restore the genome is still investigational.

Liver Disease of Pregnancy
Cholestasis of pregnancy

Cholestasis of pregnancy (intrahepatic cholestasis of pregnancy, benign recurrent cholestasis) should be treated as a high-risk pregnancy, because the disease carries some risk for the fetus, chiefly prematurity (rates vary from < 7% to 60% in different studies). Sudden fetal death occurs in 1% to 2% of cases, but is rare before the 35th week of gestation. Some authorities recommend delivery after fetal lung maturity is achieved, because fetal risk is greatest in the final month of gestation.

Symptoms and laboratory abnormalities usually resolve after delivery, although cholestasis occasionally is prolonged. Treatment before delivery is primarily symptomatic. Ursodeoxycholic acid may be helpful and is tolerated well by both the patient and the fetus. Cholestyramine can help symptoms, but worsens steatorrhea and fat-soluble vitamin malabsorption. Sedatives such as phenobarbitol or hydroxyzine (Atarax, Vistaril) may give some relief from the itching.

Acute Fatty Liver of Pregnancy

The mainstay of treatment of AFLP is prompt delivery of the fetus, with intensive care monitoring and support as the liver recovers. The intensive care unit team must be prepared to handle a variety of catastrophes, including disseminated intravascular coagulation, renal failure, respiratory failure, ascites or pleural effusions, and infections. Most patients recover completely if AFLP is diagnosed early and complications are treated aggressively.

Liver Disease of Preeclampsia and HELLP Syndrome

Liver disease of preeclampsia resolves after delivery; treatment is directed toward timely delivery of the fetus and management of the preeclampsia.

Management of HELLP syndrome is supportive, with intensive care unit observation until the baby can be safely delivered. Corticosteroids (e.g., dexamethasone [Decadron] 10 mg intravenously every 12 hours) improve laboratory abnormalities and facilitate fetal lung maturation. Severe cases may require platelet transfusion or plasmapheresis. Some patients can be safely observed without delivery if the aminotransferases and platelet abnormalities improve.

FOLLOW-UP

When a clear diagnosis emerges after a step-wise approach to a patient with elevated liver enzymes, treatment and follow-up are straightforward. A more difficult situation arises after evaluation of a patient who has no clear diagnosis after going through the appropriate diagnostic evaluation (no risk factors or family history of liver disease; the serology is negative for viral and autoimmune hepatitis; hemochromatosis is excluded; and the imaging test is normal or shows fatty liver). Fatty liver is the most common diagnosis and is not associated with any morbidity; in such cases, a liver biopsy may not be necessary. However, it is often difficult to distinguish between someone who is obese and has only fatty liver, and someone who is both obese and has another underlying liver disease.

Patients who have asymptomatic elevations of aminotransferases or alkaline phosphatase should have the enzyme levels repeated in 3 to 6 months (see algorithms).

Patient Education

Most patients with asymptomatic elevations of liver enzymes should be advised to avoid hepatotoxic medications and reduce or eliminate alcohol consumption. Environmental toxins should also be removed. Further treatment and advice depend on the specific findings of the workup. If elevated liver enzymes persist with no definitive diagnosis, the patient should be reassured, but periodic recheck of the enzyme levels is prudent.

Patients at risk should be encouraged to receive vaccines for hepatitis A or hepatitis B. The Advisory Committee on Immunization Practices (ACIP) now recommends immunization of children in geographic areas with consistently elevated rates of hepatitis A.

SUGGESTED READING

Anderson PB. Liver dysfunction. In: Reilly BM, ed. *Practical strategies in outpatient medicine*, 2nd ed. Philadelphia: WB Saunders, 1991.

Bacon BR, Powell LW, Adams PC, et al. Molecular medicine and hemochromatosis: at the crossroads. *Gastroenterology* 1999;116:193-207.

Bacq Y. Intrahepatic cholestasis of pregnancy. *Clinics in Liver Disease* 1999;3:1-13.

Bates B, Yellin JA. The yield of multiphasic screening. *JAMA* 1972;222:74-78.

Catalina G, Navarro V. Hepatitis C: a challenge for the generalist. *Hosp Pract (Off Ed)* 2000;24:97-118.

Cebul RD, Beck JF. Biochemical profiles: applications in ambulatory screening and preadmission testing of adults. *Ann Intern Med* 1987;106:403-413.

Feldman M, ed. *Sleisenger and Fordtran's gastrointestinal and liver disease*, 6th ed. Philadelphia: WB Saunders, 1998.

Fregia A, Jensen DM. Evaluation of abnormal liver tests. *Compr Ther* 1994;20:50-54.

Goddard CJR, Warnes TW. Raised liver enzymes in asymptomatic patients: investigation and outcome. *Dig Dis* 1992;10:218-226.

Gopal D, Rosen H. Abnormal findings on liver function tests. *Postgrad Med* 2000;107: 100-114.

Gordon S. Antiviral therapy for chronic hepatitis B and C. *Postgrad Med* 2000; 107:135-144.

Hay JE, Czaja AJ, Rakela J, Ludwig J. The nature of unexplained chronic aminotransferase elevations of a mild to moderate degree in asymptomatic patients. *Hepatology* 1989;9:193-197.

Hultcrantz R, Gabrielsson N. Patients with persistent elevation of aminotransferases: investigation with ultrasonography, radionuclide imaging and liver biopsy. *J Intern Med* 1993;233:7-12.

Hultcrantz R, Glaumann H, Lindberg G, Nilsson LH. Liver investigation in 149 asymptomatic patients with moderately elevated activities of serum aminotransferases. *Scand J Gastroenterol* 1986;21:109-113.

Johnston DE. Special considerations in interpreting liver function tests. *Am Fam Physician* 1999;59:2223-2230.

Kamath PS. Clinical approach to the patient with abnormal liver test results. *Mayo Clin Proc* 1996;71:1089-1095.

King PD. Abnormal liver enzyme levels. Evaluation in asymptomatic patients. *Postgrad Med* 1991;89:137-141.

Kools AM, Bloomer JR. Abnormal liver function tests. How to assess their importance in asymptomatic patients. *Postgrad Med* 1987;81:45-50.

Mayfield D, McLeod G, Hall P. The CAGE questionnaire: validation of a new alcoholism screening instrument. *Am J Psychiatry* 1974;131:1121-1123.

McDonnell SM, Witte D. Hereditary hemochromatosis. Preventing chronic effects of this underdiagnosed disorder. *Postgrad Med* 1997;102:83-94.

Morrison E, Kowdley K. Genetic liver disease in adults. *Postgrad Med* 2000;107:147-159.

Moseley RH. Approach to the patient with abnormal liver chemistries. In: Yamada T, Alpers DH, Laine L, Owyang C, Powell DW, eds. *Textbook of gastroenterology*, 3rd ed. Philadelphia: Lippincott Williams & Wilkins, 1999:946-965.

Moseley RH. Evaluation of abnormal liver function tests. *Med Clin North Am* 1996; 80:887-906.

Moyer LA, Mast EE, Alter MJ. Hepatitis C: Part II. Prevention counseling and medical evaluation. *Am Fam Physician* 1999;59:349-354, 357.

Padden MO. HELLP syndrome: recognition and perinatal management. *Am Fam Physician* 1999;60:829-839.

Rosalki SB, Dooley JS. Liver function profiles and their interpretation. *Br J Hosp Med* 1994;1444-1448.

Theal RM, Scott K. Evaluating asymptomatic patients with abnormal liver function test results. *Am Fam Physician* 1996;53:2111-2119.

Van Ness MM, Diehl AM. Is liver biopsy useful in the evaluation of patients with chronically elevated liver enzymes? *Ann Intern Med* 1989;111:473-478.

Wolf J. Liver disease in pregnancy. *Med Clin North Am* 1996;80:1167-1187.

Yamada T, Alpers DH, Laine L, Owyang C, Powell DW, eds. *Textbook of gastroenterology*, 3rd ed. Philadelphia: Lippincott Williams & Wilkns, 1999.

Younossi ZM. Evaluating asymptomatic patients with mildly elevated liver enzymes. *Clev Clin J Med* 1998;65:150-158.

CHAPTER 6

....

Gastrointestinal Disorders in Pregnancy

Mark C. Potter

DEFINITION

Gastrointestinal (GI) symptoms are so common in pregnancy that they are expected by both pregnant women and their physicians. Occasionally, serious GI disorders must be diagnosed and managed during pregnancy. The challenge to physicians is to minimize risk to the fetus by choosing the safest possible diagnostic tests and therapies. This chapter reviews GI disorders that complicate pregnancy and recommends the least risky evaluation and management. Within each section of this chapter, conditions will be discussed in order from the mouth to the rectum.

CLINICAL MANIFESTATIONS

Gingivitis is common in pregnancy, but it is not caused by pregnancy. Pregnant women's gums become more hyperemic and can bleed more easily. Pregnancy should result in no increase in gum disease or caries if good oral hygiene is observed.

Heartburn, or gastroesophageal reflux disease (GERD), affects between 30% and 80% of pregnant women, which is significantly higher than in age-matched controls. The incidence of GERD increases with each trimester. Symptoms are the same as in nonpregnant persons, including burning discomfort in the midepigastrium or central chest. Severe symptoms or lack of response to standard management (described below) should prompt consideration of peptic ulcer or biliary or pancreatic disease.

Nausea is experienced by 60% to 90% and vomiting by 40% to 50% of pregnant women. These symptoms most often begin during the 6th week from the last menstrual period and resolve between the 14th and 20th week. Of pregnant women, 1% to 2% experience nausea and vomiting throughout pregnancy. If the pattern or severity of nausea or vomiting is atypical, more serious GI disease must be considered (Table 6.1).

Abdominal pain is not associated with common "morning sickness" and requires the physician to search for a cause, either gastrointestinal or obstetric (Table 6.2).

Hyperemesis gravidarum is an uncommon condition affecting 0.3% to 1% of pregnancies, in which intractable nausea and vomiting result in dehydration, electrolyte abnormalities, and weight loss.

Peptic ulcer disease (PUD) during pregnancy presents with the same symptoms as in nonpregnant patients. Typically, this includes gnawing epigastric pain, which may radiate to the back and may be alleviated by eating. PUD is less common in pregnant women than in age-matched controls.

Pancreatitis presents similarly in both pregnant and nonpregnant patients, with constant epigastric pain often with nausea and vomiting. Pancreatitis complicates 0.01% to 0.1% of pregnancies.

TABLE 6.1. Differential diagnosis of nausea, vomiting, and abdominal pain in pregnancy

	Abdominal pain	History	Physical examination	Laboratory	Ultrasound	Abdominal x-ray
Morning sickness	Absent	Subacute First trimester	Normal	Normal	Normal	Normal
Hyperemesis	Absent	Subacute First trimester	Distressed Dehydrated	Electrolyte depletion	Normal	Normal
Peptic ulcer disease or gastritis	Present	Subacute, relieved by food Prior PUD	Midepigastric tenderness	Normal, or anemic if bleeding	Normal	Normal
Biliary or gallbladder disease	Present	Acute or recurrent	Right upper quadrant tenderness	Increased GGT, ALP	Distention, stones, sludge	Stones usually radiolucent Possible ileus
Liver disease	Present	Viral: infection risk IHCP: itch, subacute HELLP: malaise AFLP: fulminant, delirium, shock	Jaundice Right upper quadrant tenderness	See Table 6.3	HELLP: may show hemorrhage AFLP: fatty infiltration	Normal
Appendicitis	Present	Acute onset, anorexia. Pain may be in flank or upper abdomen in later pregnancy.	Right sided abdominal or flank tenderness, muted peritoneal signs	Often moderate neutrophil elevation	Normal, or fluid around appendix	Possible ileus
Intestinal obstruction	Present	Acute, with relatively muted pain Vomiting and constipation follow	Muted peritoneal signs Decreased bowel tones	Normal early; later, neutrophil elevation	Normal	Dilated bowel, air fluid levels

AFLP, acute fatty liver of pregnancy; ALP, alkaline phosphatase; GGT, gamma-glutamyltransferase; HELLP, hemolysis, elevated liver enzymes, low platelets; IHCP, intrahepatic cholestasis of pregnancy; PUD, peptic ulcer disease.

T ABLE 6.2. Causes of acute abdomen in pregnancy

NONOBSTETRIC CAUSES
Acute appendicitis
Acute cholecystitis
Acute pancreatitis
Hepatic rupture
Intestinal obstruction
Adnexal torsion
Sickle cell crisis

OBSTETRIC CAUSES
Ectopic pregnancy
Abruptio placentae
Red degeneration of a uterine myoma
Uterine rupture

From Zimmermann EM, Christman GM. Approach to Gastrointestinal disease in the female patient. In: Yamada T, Alpers DH, Laine L, Owyang C, Powell DW, eds. *Textbook of gastroenterology*, 3rd ed. Philadelphia: Lippincott Williams & Wilkins, 1999:1066.

Acute intestinal obstruction presents in pregnancy with the classic triad of abdominal pain, emesis, and constipation, but the frequency of these complaints in normal pregnancy often results in delayed diagnosis. Further complicating the diagnosis of intestinal obstruction are the enlarged uterus, normally elevated white blood cell count, and risk associated with abdominal x-ray studies. Adhesions from prior surgery appear to be the inciting cause in at least 50% of cases, and a high index of suspicion must be maintained when evaluating patients with abdominal scars. Of pregnancies, 1 of 1,500 to 3,500 are affected by adhesions from prior surgery.

The liver is subject to three conditions unique to pregnancy: intrahepatic cholestasis of pregnancy (IHCP), acute fatty liver of pregnancy (AFLP), and HELLP syndrome. IHCP is an idiopathic disorder of the second and third trimesters whose hallmark is itching, especially of the palms and soles, especially at night. Malaise and anorexia are common. All symptoms increase until delivery, then rapidly decline. Abdominal pain and hepatomegaly should be absent.

A more acute and far more dangerous condition is AFLP— which is idiopathic true liver failure. AFLP is heralded by nausea, vomiting, and abdominal pain. This is followed in 1 to 2 weeks by jaundice, confusion, and bleeding. AFLP will progress, if untreated, to coma and death. Of pregnancies, 1 of 10,000 are affected by AFLP, with a maternal and fetal mortality rate of approximately 25%. HELLP syndrome and preeclampsia are present in 30% to 100% of cases.

The HELLP syndrome is composed of hemolysis, elevated liver enzymes, and low platelets. It is one of the spectrum of related diseases that includes preeclampsia and AFLP. HELLP syndrome occurs in 20% of patients with preeclampsia, or 0.25% to 1% of all pregnancies. Signs of preeclampsia, however, may be absent in 8% to 15% of cases of HELLP syndrome. Clinical manifestations include malaise (90%), right upper quadrant pain (81%), and headache (36%). When hypertension is absent, diagnosis requires a high index of suspicion. Any nonspecific illness in late pregnancy, a platelet count of less than 150,000, or evidence of hemolysis should raise the suspicion of HELLP syndrome.

Viral hepatitis presents with abdominal pain, malaise, and jaundice. The presentation and course of viral hepatitis are not significantly altered by pregnancy. Exceptions to this rule are hepatitis E and herpes simplex virus that may be fulminant and lead to liver necrosis. Patients with symptoms of liver disease and lesions suggestive of herpes simplex virus should be rapidly evaluated, as treatment with acyclovir is effective.

Acute cholecystitis and biliary colic may be slightly more common during pregnancy. The clinical presentation, which is unaltered by pregnancy, includes right upper quadrant pain, nausea, and vomiting. A history of previous biliary colic or fatty food intolerance is present in 80% of cases. Cholecystitis in pregnancy is rare, affecting 1 of 1,000 to 1 of 10,000 live births.

The clinical presentation of acute appendicitis is significantly altered by pregnancy. A progressive displacement of the appendix occurs upward and rightward during the second and third trimesters (Figure 6.1). The abdominal pain and tenderness

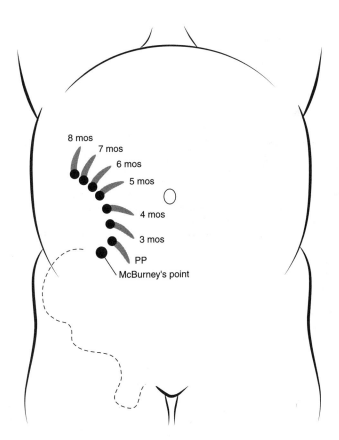

FIGURE 6.1. Change in the position of the appendix during pregnancy. PP, postpartum. (From Clark Hill W, Fleming AD. Gastrointestinal diseases complicating pregnancy. In: Reece EA, Hobbins JC, eds. *Medicine of the fetus and mother*, 2nd ed. Philadelphia: Lippincott Williams & Wilkins, 1999:1135.)

of appendicitis are often reduced, which can delay diagnosis. Thus, peritonitis is present in 50% of cases by the time surgery is performed.

Inflammatory bowel disease (ulcerative colitis and Crohn's disease) is unaffected in frequency or course by pregnancy. Exacerbations present with crampy abdominal pain and loose or bloody stools. The risk of fetal loss is related to disease activity and is not increased when disease is quiescent.

Constipation is reported by between 11% and 40% of pregnant women, with occurrence increasing by trimester. However, 25% of age-matched controls have reported constipation, and laxative use is reported by a greater number of nonpregnant women. Complaints include decreased stool frequency, more difficulty passing stool, and hard stools.

Hemorrhoids are more common in pregnancy, in later trimesters, and in each subsequent pregnancy. Manifestations include itching, bleeding, and pain.

PHYSICAL EXAMINATION

The physical examination related to gastroenterologic disease in pregnancy is in most ways the same as outside of pregnancy. Certain parts of the examination warrant specific mention, however. Careful blood pressure monitoring, and looking for jaundice and petechiae may uncover liver disease. Abdominal examination is complicated by the presence of the enlarged uterus. The liver is displaced upward and posteriorly, so that a palpable liver edge strongly suggests enlargement. The appendix is progressively displaced upward and laterally as described. Peritoneal signs are reduced, including rebound and guarding. The abdomen and uterus should not be tender in normal pregnancy. Lower extremity edema is normal in later pregnancy, but nondependent edema, especially with rapid weight gain, suggests preeclampsia.

DIAGNOSTIC STUDIES

The primary impact of pregnancy on studies is on the use of radiology. A safe dose of x-rays in pregnancy has not been determined. Commonly cited is the work of Brent, who determined that approximately 10 Rads are needed to induce congenital defects. An abdominal plain film exposes the fetus to 290 mRad and a barium enema to 800 mRad. Exposure to 1 Rad was associated with a malformation risk of 0.1%. Major malformations are unlikely below 5 Rads. Fetal x-ray exposure should be minimized but should not prevent the use of x-ray when needed [e.g., to diagnose bowel obstruction or for endoscopic retrograde cholangiopancreatography (ERCP) in the setting of a common bile duct stone].

The esophagus, stomach, and duodenum can be evaluated by endoscopy, which is considered safe in pregnancy.

Ultrasound is considered safe in pregnancy and is the modality of choice to evaluate the gallbladder and biliary tree.

Laboratory tests with elevated levels in pregnancy include alkaline phosphatase (up to a fourfold elevation), lipids, and fibrinogen. Albumin is decreased (by 20%), as is gamma-globulin. Tests that are unaffected by pregnancy include coagulation studies, bilirubin, and transaminases.

RISK FACTORS

Nausea and vomiting are more commonly reported by younger women, primiparas, nonsmokers, and housewives. Hyperemesis gravidarum is more common among primiparas and overweight women, and in twin pregnancies.

Peptic ulcer disease risk factors are those of the general population, including cigarette smoking, nonsteroidal antiinflammatory drug use, and *Helicobacter pylori* infection.

Cholelithiasis is more common among women with pregnancies before age 25 years, more than four pregnancies, and increased weight.

Pancreatitis risk factors include gallstones (which cause 90% of pancreatitis in pregnancy), excessive alcohol use, and familial hypertriglyceridemia, which is occasionally unmasked by the physiologic rise in triglycerides in the third trimester.

The primary risk factor for intestinal obstruction is prior abdominal or pelvic surgery or infection.

Intrahepatic cholestasis of pregnancy is more common in Chile, Scandinavia, and the Middle East, in the fall and winter, and in those with a family history.

Acute fatty liver of pregnancy often overlaps with HELLP, whose risk factors are those of preeclampsia: nulliparity, extremes of age, and twin gestation.

Risk factors for viral hepatitis are the same in pregnancy as outside of pregnancy (e.g., parenteral blood exposure, or contaminated water consumption).

PATHOPHYSIOLOGY

During pregnancy, circulating blood volume increases, as does cardiac output. These changes have been invoked to explain gingival hyperplasia and the increased incidence of hemorrhoids in pregnancy.

Progesterone has been shown to reduce smooth muscle tone in animals. This effect is thought to contribute to reduced lower esophageal sphincter tone, which may account for the recognized increase in GERD during pregnancy. This smooth muscle relaxation may also explain a demonstrated increase in intestinal transit time. Increased transit time, compression of the colon by the uterus, and increased sodium reabsorption by the colon are thought to underlie constipation in pregnancy.

The pathophysiology of gallstones in pregnancy includes increased lithogenicity of the bile produced and reduced gallbladder contractility.

The primary liver disorders of pregnancy—IHCP, AFLP, and HELLP syndrome—are idiopathic. In IHCP, impairment of bile acid secretion is the most prominent defect. In AFLP, hepatocyte and portal system destruction takes place. In HELLP syndrome, microvascular injury with microinfarction involves the liver.

DIFFERENTIAL DIAGNOSIS

A full differential diagnosis of all gastrointestinal disorders possible during pregnancy is beyond the scope of this chapter. Differential diagnoses for the most common and the most serious conditions are presented here. For the differential diagnoses of nausea, vomiting, and abdominal pain see Table 6.1. For the differential diagnosis of abnormal liver tests see Table 6.3.

A differential diagnosis of abdominal pain in pregnancy must include the causes of acute abdomen listed in Table 6.2, as well as the full differential of abdominal pain outside of pregnancy (see Chapter 1). Conditions unique to pregnancy that cause abdominal pain, or in which pregnancy significantly alters the evaluation of abdominal pain are discussed below.

Upper abdominal pain can be caused by GERD, PUD, gastritis, liver or biliary disease, pancreatitis, or appendicitis in late pregnancy. When symptoms are mild, careful history and physical examination are often adequate to guide an initial therapeutic trial (e.g., antacids or dietary advice for GERD). Further evaluation, if indicated, should include a complete blood cell count, serum transaminases, alkaline phosphatase, bilirubin, and lipase or amylase levels. Differentiating between liver diseases in preg-

T ABLE 6.3. Differential diagnosis of abnormal liver tests in pregnancy

	Presentation	Diagnostics
Intrahepatic cholestasis of pregnancy (IHCP)	Itch, jaundice, pain absent, usually after 30 wks	Increased conjugated bilirubin, mildly increased liver enzymes
Acute fatty liver of pregnancy (AFLP)	Fulminant illness, jaundice, nausea and vomiting, encephalopathy, shock Late third trimester	Increased liver enzymes, bilirubin, d-dimer, uric acid, neutrophils Decreased platelets, fibrinogen, glucose
Viral hepatitis	Jaundice, mild pain, itch	Increased transaminases, bilirubin Virus-specific serology
HELLP syndrome	Malaise, abdominal pain, usually with PIH signs and symptoms	Hemolysis, decreased haptoglobin Increased liver enzymes, d-dimer Decreased platelets, fibrinogen
Biliary and gallbladder disease	Pain, fever if infected	Increased transaminases, GGT Abnormal ultrasound

GGT, gamma-glutamyltransferase; HELLP, hemolysis, elevated liver enzymes, low platelets; PIH, pregnancy-induced hypertension.

nancy relies on viral serologies, the serum tests listed above, and ultrasound and x-ray studies, as described below. Liver biopsy can be performed during pregnancy when a diagnosis cannot be made by any other means.

IHCP presents with itching and elevated bile salts, of which cholylglycine is the most widely tested for. Transaminases are moderately elevated, four to ten times control. Bilirubin is rarely above 3 mg/dl.

In AFLP, serum alkaline phosphatase, transaminases, bilirubin, uric acid, and creatinine are almost always elevated. Disseminated intravascular coagulation and coagulopathy occur in 50% of cases. Serum glucose may be dangerously low. A very high neutrophil count may distinguish this from acute viral hepatitis, HELLP syndrome, or thrombotic thrombocytopenic purpura. Hemolysis is uncommon in AFLP, which is also distinct from HELLP syndrome. A liver biopsy demonstrating microvesicular fat provides a definitive diagnosis.

In HELLP syndrome, intravascular hemolysis is present with red blood cell fragments and schistocytes visible on a peripheral blood smear. Haptoglobin is low. A platelet count below 150,000 and moderately elevated transaminases are typical. Serum creatinine and uric acid are usually elevated. The presence of d-dimer may precede the typical drop in fibrinogen. Prolonged prothrombin and partial thromboplastin time are relatively late findings.

Appendicitis must be diagnosed clinically, although ultrasound and complete blood cell count findings may help in some cases. The classic physical findings of point tenderness and peritonitis are often blunted. Nausea, emesis, and anorexia may be falsely attributed to pregnancy itself or to upper abdominal pathology in later pregnancy.

REFERRAL

Any suggestion of surgical disease, such as appendicitis or obstruction, should prompt early consultation or referral. Dental surgery with local anesthetic is considered safe, and urgent dental procedures should not be delayed. Workup of moderate liver enzyme elevations can be undertaken by family physicians in stable patients as described above.

Evidence of AFLP, HELLP syndrome, or brisk GI bleeding are emergencies requiring intensive obstetric care, preferably in a tertiary center, and preparation for urgent delivery.

MANAGEMENT

Medication safety in pregnancy must always include a careful review of the known and potential risks, weighed against expected benefits. In 1979, the US Food and Drug Administration (FDA) established the following commonly cited five categories of possible adverse effects of drugs on the fetus.

Category A: Controlled studies in humans have demonstrated no fetal risk (e.g., multivitamins at recommended daily allowances).

Category B: Animal studies have demonstrated no risk and human studies are lacking, or animal studies demonstrated risk but controlled human studies did not.

Category C: No adequate animal or human studies are available, or risk was found in animal studies but no controlled human studies are available.

Category D: Known risks to human fetuses, but in which benefit may outweigh risk (e.g., phenytoin or carbamazepine).

Category X: Known risks that clearly outweigh any benefit (e.g., warfarin).

Gastrointestinal medications that are often used in pregnancy are described in Table 6.4 and below.

Regarding gingivitis and tooth decay, good oral hygiene should be actively encouraged. Elective dental surgery should be scheduled, when needed, for the second trimester.

Nausea and vomiting, without dehydration or electrolyte abnormalities, have no negative impact on pregnancy outcomes. Medical management must, therefore, weigh possible fetal risk against maternal discomfort. No FDA-approved treatments are available for control of nausea and vomiting in pregnancy. Bendectin, a combination of pyridoxine (vitamin B_6) and doxylamine, was withdrawn from the market by the manufacturer because of legal action, but teratogenicity has not been clearly demonstrated. Vitamin B_6 (25 mg by mouth every 8 hours) has been demonstrated to be more effective than placebo, but this regimen, which exceeds the US recommended dietary allowance, is rated category C. Among antiemetics, meclizine (Antivert) and metoclopramide (Reglan) are category B, and are not FDA approved for use in pregnancy. Nonpharmacologic measures that can help reduce nausea and vomiting include eating small frequent meals and avoiding strong food odors. Hyperemesis gravidarum often requires intravenous hydration and antiemetics. Psychosocial evaluation is indicated and psychosocial interventions have demonstrated efficacy.

Heartburn, or GERD, should first be managed by avoiding large, fatty, or spicy meals, and not eating immediately before going to bed. Failing this, oral antacids usually are adequate and are considered to be the safest medical treatment. Histamine$_2$ (H_2) blockers, if necessary, may be effective. Ranitidine (Zantac) is probably safest, but despite its category B rating, large studies of H_2 blockers in pregnancy are lacking and this class of drugs is not considered to be safe for routine use in pregnancy. Proton pump inhibitors should be reserved for known refractory esophagitis or ulcer disease.

IHCP is a very challenging management problem, which focuses on alleviating itch and preventing fetal loss. Cholestyramine (Questran; category C; 4 g four to five times per day) helps 50% of cases. Fat-soluble vitamin malabsorption can occur. Prothrombin time must be monitored and elevations treated with vitamin K. Phenobarbital (category D) has also been reported to reduce itching by 50%. Increased rates of fetal loss, prematurity, and postpartum hemorrhage have been associated with IHCP, and

T ABLE 6.4.   Commonly used gastrointestinal drugs in pregnancy and lactation

	Animal studies of fertility	Pregnancy category	Present in breast milk
Acid-Lowering Drugs			
Antacids	Not studied	Considered safe[a]	Unknown
Cimetidine (Tagamet)	No known effect	B[b]	Y
Ranitidine (Zantac)	No known effect	B	Y
Famotidine (Pepcid)	No known effect	B	Y
Nizatidine (Axid)	No known effect	B	Y
Sucralfate (Carafate)	No known effect	B	Minimal
Omeprazole (Prilosec)	No known effect	C—embryo/fetal toxicity	Unknown
Lansoprazole (Prevacid)	No known effect	B	Y
Antiemetics			
Meclizine (Antivert)	Not studied	B	Unknown
Diphenhydramine (Benadryl)	No known effect	B	Y
Promethazine (Phenergan)	Not studied	C	Unknown
Prochlorperazine (Compazine)	Not studied	C[c]	Unknown
Antidiarrheals			
Diphenoxylate/atropine (Lomotil)	Decreased fertility	C	Y
Loperamide (Imodium-AD)	No known effect	B	Unknown
Attapulgite (Kaopectate)	Not studied[d]	None available	Unknown
Bismuth subsalicylate (Pepto-Bismol)	Not studied	C (1st, 2nd trimester), D (3rd trimester)	Unknown
Laxatives			
Psyllium (Metamucil)			
Citrucil	No known effect	B	Unknown
Magnesium hydroxide (Milk of Magnesia)	No known effect	Considered safe	Unknown
	No known effect	B	Unknown
Bisacodyl (Dulcolax)	No known effect	B	Unknown
Docusate sodium	No known effect	C	Unknown
Promotility Agents			
Metoclopramide (Reglan)	[e]	B	Y
Antispasmotics			
Dicyclomine (Bentyl)	No known effect	B	Unknown
Donnatal	Not studied	C—not studied	Unknown
Hyoscyamine (Levsin)	Not studied	C—not studied	Unknown

continued

T ABLE 6.4 *continued*. Commonly used gastrointestinal drugs in pregnancy and lactation

	Animal studies of fertility	Pregnancy category	Present in breast milk
Inflammatory Bowel Disease Drugs			
Sulfasalazine[f] (Azulfidine)	Decreased fertility	B[g]	Y[g]
Prednisone	No known effect	B	Y
Mesalamine			
Asacol	No known effect	B	Y
Pentasa	No known effect	B	Y
Rowasa	No known effect	B	Y
Azathioprine (Imuran)	Decreased fertility	D	Unknown
Metronidazole (Flagyl)	No known effect	B[h]	Y
Cyclosporine (Sardimmune)	No known effect	C	Y

[a]Antacids are considered safe in low doses. Cases of hypercalcemia, hyper- and hypomagnesemia, and tendon hyperreflexia in fetuses and neonates of mothers on high doses of aluminum, calcium, or magnesium antacids have been identified.

[b]Antiandrogen effect in male litter dams.

[c]Prolonged jaundice, extrapyramidal side effects, hyperreflexia, or hyporeflexia in newborn infants whose mothers received phenothiazines.

[d]Safety not studied: however, minimal Kaopectate is absorbed systemically so little systemic toxicity is expected.

[e]Increases prolactin levels; clinical significance is unknown.

[f]Reversible oligospermia and infertility in men treated with sulfasalazine.

[g]Sulfonamides displace bilirubin and may cause kernicterus.

[h]Tumorigenic in mice and rats; no effects on fertility or fetus in animal studies.

Category A, controlled human studies failed to demonstrate a risk to the fetus and the possibility of fetal harm appears remote.

Category B, Either animal studies have not demonstrated a fetal risk but there are no controlled studies in pregnant women, or animal studies have shown an adverse effect that was not confirmed in controlled human studies.

Category C, Either studies in animals have revealed adverse effects on the fetus and there are no controlled studies in women, or studies in women and animals are not available.

Category D, There is evidence of human fetal risk.

From Briggs GG, Freeman RK, Yaffe SJ, eds. *Drugs in pregnancy and lactation*, 5th ed. Baltimore: Williams & Wilkins; 1998.

From Zimmermann EM, Christman GM. Approach to gastrointestinal disease in the female patient. In: Yamada T, Alpers DH, Laine L, Owyang C, Powell DW, eds. *Textbook of Gastroenterology*, 3rd ed. Philadelphia: Lippincott Williams & Wilkins, 1999:1063.

NOTE: It is recommended that current information be verified prior to prescribing drugs for pregnant patients.

elective delivery at fetal lung maturity has been advocated by some. Close monitoring of fetal well-being is recommended.

Management of HELLP syndrome begins with assessment of severity, for which the platelet count and lactate dehydrogenase levels are the best markers. Consultation should be obtained, and magnesium sulfate seizure prophylaxis should be started. The patient should be transferred to a center with neonatal services appropriate to the gestational age of the fetus. In mild cases, before 34 weeks of gestation, consider treatment with corticosteroids and close monitoring. In moderate cases, consider inducing labor with the goal of delivery within 48 hours. In severe cases or gestation less than 32 weeks, a caesarean section is indicated.

Management of AFLP should be done at a tertiary center with neonatology and perinatology services available. Initial management must include stabilization of shock, treatment of hypoglycemia, and correction of coagulopathy.

Management of biliary colic and acute cholecystitis in pregnancy is controversial. Complicating the diagnosis are the increased rates of gallstones and biliary sludge in pregnant women (11% and 33%, respectively). Conservative management (bowel rest, intravenous fluids, analgesics, and antibiotics) is effective in 77% to 84% of cases. If elective cholecystectomy is chosen, the second trimester is considered the safest, during which period fetal loss has been reported at 5%.

Management of constipation in pregnancy should begin with instructions to the patient on adequate dietary fiber and fluid intake. If medications are to be used, fiber supplements [e.g., psyllium (Metamucil, Fiberall)], or magnesium hydroxide (milk of magnesia) are considered safe by many physicians.

FOLLOW-UP

Most physicians practicing obstetrics follow pregnant patients more closely than they do other patients with comparable conditions. This extra attentiveness is warranted, as injury to the fetus can lead to an entire lifetime of consequences. Appropriate follow-up begins with appropriate education of each pregnant woman about what changes are considered normal to pregnancy, and what warning signs to watch for. Many women know that they may experience morning sickness, heartburn, abdominal discomfort, fatigue, changes in bowel habits, and hemorrhoids. Every pregnant patient should be counseled to report promptly signs of dehydration, severe vomiting, and all moderate or severe abdominal pain. Instructions should be given to report nondependent edema, rapid gain in weight, significantly increased headache, and moderate or severe malaise. Once abnormal symptoms or signs have been identified, close follow-up to resolution or prompt and systematic evaluation must be undertaken.

Evaluation of GI problems in pregnancy is an everyday activity for family physicians who practice obstetrics, but when serious problems arise and are handled correctly, it can be of tremendous benefit to two patients at once during a critical life stage.

SUGGESTED READING

Brent RL. The effects of embryonic and fetal exposure to x-ray, microwaves and ultrasound. *Clin Obstet Gynecol* 1983;26:484.

Burrow GN, Ferris TF, eds. *Medical complications during pregnancy*, 4th ed. Philadelphia: WB Saunders, 1995.

Creasy R, Resnide R. *Maternal-fetal medicine: principles and practice*, 3rd ed. Philadelphia: WB Saunders, 1994.

Gastrointestinal disease: pathophysiology/diagnosis/management, 6th ed. Philadelphia: WB Saunders, 1998.

Padden MO. HELLP syndrome: recognition and perinatal management. *Am Fam Physician* 1999;60(3):829–836.

Reese EA, Hobbins JC, Mahoney MJ. *Medicine of the fetus and mother*. Philadelphia: JB Lippincott, 1992.

Zimmermann EM, Christman GM. Approach to gastrointestinal disease in the female patient. In: Yamada T, Alpers DH, Laine L, Owyang C, Powell DW, eds. *Textbook of gastroenterology*, 3rd ed. Philadelphia: Lippincott Williams & Wilkins; 1999: 1059–1080.

CHAPTER 7

Biliary Colic

Arlene Sagan

DEFINITION

Biliary colic is a steady, severe pain usually in the right upper quadrant of the abdomen caused by obstruction of the cystic duct. Gallstone disease is by far the most common cause of biliary colic, although a tumor or stricture can cause similar symptoms.

CLINICAL MANIFESTATIONS

Biliary colic is common. Gallstones develop in approximately 50% of women and 20% of men by age 75 years. Gallstones can be asymptomatic (incidentally found during an evaluation for another problem) or they can cause a single episode or recurrent episodes of biliary colic. Gallstones also cause complications such as acute cholecystitis, cholangitis, or acute pancreatitis. The family physician must distinguish between patients with symptoms caused by gallstones and those with silent stones and abdominal pain attributable to dyspepsia or other nonbiliary causes (Table 7.1).

PATIENT HISTORY

The initial history should elicit the location, duration, and character of the pain. Biliary colic is sudden in onset, building to a maximum within 1 hour. The pain is not "colicky" or paroxysmal but rather constant and severe, generally lasting 2 to 6 hours.

T ABLE 7.1. Signs and symptoms helpful in the diagnosis of biliary colic and acute cholecystitis

Finding	Biliary colic	Acute cholecystitis
Location of pain	RUQ	RUQ
Quality of pain	Severe, steady	Severe, steady; return of pain
Peritoneal signs	No	Yes
Nausea/vomiting	Uncommon	Common
Jaundice/elevated bilirubin	Rare	Common
Fever	No	Common to 101°F
Palpable gallbladder	No	Yes in 50% of cases
Rigid abdomen	No	Common
Elevated WBC	No	Common
Usual treatment	Elective laparoscopic cholecystectomy	Urgent laparoscopic cholecystectomy

RUQ, right upper quadrant; WBC, white blood cell count.

93

It is generally localized to the right upper quadrant (RUQ) or epigastrium and can radiate to the left or right scapula.

Symptoms are almost always infrequent, with weeks to months passing between episodes. Symptoms tend to occur when the patient is in bed with the gallbladder horizontal and the stones are closer to the opening of the cystic duct. Biliary colic can occur after eating a fatty meal as the bile flow moves a small stone into the cystic duct.

An attack of biliary pain is not relieved by taking over-the-counter medications, changing position, or defecating. Vomiting can occur. Belching and bloating are not problems attributable to gallstone disease.

Biliary colic usually subsides within 6 hours because the stone that caused the attack has either dropped back into the gallbladder or has passed out of the common bile duct. If the stone does not pass from the cystic duct, then acute cholecystitis (inflammation of the gallbladder outlet) can occur.

PHYSICAL EXAMINATION

A patient with biliary colic typically presents with readily apparent, unrelenting, severe RUQ discomfort. The presence of fever or abdominal rigidity when the pain passes suggests acute cholecystitis or local peritonitis. Murphy's sign (involuntary cessation of inspiration because of deep palpation beneath the right costal arch, below the hepatic margin) is often seen with acute cholecystitis (Table 7.1).

DIAGNOSTIC STUDIES

Biliary colic needs to be differentiated from more severe gallstone complications. Initial studies include hemoglobin, a white blood cell (WBC) count with differential, liver function tests, amylase, and ultrasonography of the RUQ. Laboratory abnormalities are uncommon in persons with simple biliary colic. Abnormal results suggest a complication of gallstone obstruction or a nonbiliary diagnosis. Gallstones can be easily identified on ultrasound. Determining whether a patient's symptoms are attributable to gallstones is the diagnostic challenge.

Ultrasound is the optimal technique to identify gallstones. Ultrasound is very accurate, with sensitivity and specificity of more than 95%. It allows simultaneous scanning of the gallbladder, liver, bile ducts, and pancreas. It is not limited by jaundice or pregnancy. Stones as small as 2 mm in diameter can be identified. Ultrasound also identifies biliary sludge, a precursor form of gallstones. Other causes of abdominal pain that can mimic biliary colic, (e.g., pancreatitis) may also be detected. Ultrasound testing is limited diagnostically in patients with ascites or excessive bowel gas, obese patients, and those who have had a recent barium study.

Radioisotope scans [i.e., hepatobiliary radionuclide scans (Tc-HIDA)] are useful to confirm a suspected case of acute cholecystitis, including acalculous cholecystitis. The isotype is injected intravenously, taken up by the liver, and excreted into the bile. Images are obtained 1 hour later. The gallbladder, common bile duct, and duodenum are visualized in 60 minutes in the normal patient. Persistent nonvisualization of the gallbladder (with the common bile duct and duodenum visualized) is characteristic of acute cholecystitis. Delayed visualization can occur with chronic cholecystitis.

Oral cholecystography has largely been replaced by ultrasound and radioisotope scans. However, it is still used for those patients considering nonsurgical treatments (e.g., lithotripsy or bile acid dissolution therapy.) The evening before the study, the patient fasts after a light supper and swallows the radiocontrast tablets. In a fasting patient, the dye is concentrated within the gallbladder if the cystic duct is patent and the gallbladder is functioning. A fluoroscope is then used to determine the size, composition, and number of stones.

Plain abdominal films may detect gallstones containing sufficient calcium to be radiopaque. The films are low in cost and widely available, but their primary usefulness is in the diagnosis of gallbladder complications, such as porcelain gallbladder, emphysematous cholecystitis, and gallstone ileus.

RISK FACTORS

Risk factors for gallstone formation are listed in Table 7.2.

PATHOPHYSIOLOGY

Bile formed in the liver is collected in the common hepatic duct, which joins the cystic duct of the gallbladder to form the common bile duct (CBD). The CBD descends behind the duodenum, then joins with the main pancreatic duct to empty into the duodenum at the duodenal papilla (Vater's ampulla). A stone lodged in the cystic duct causes biliary colic or acute cholecystitis. A stone lodged in the CBD leads to obstructive jaundice, cholangitis, or acute gallstone pancreatitis. A stone too large to pass into the cystic duct can gradually form a fistula from the body of the gallbladder to the duodenum or hepatic flexure of the colon. A large stone can then pass into the bowel lumen and cause acute intestinal obstruction (gallstone ileus). The severe pain experienced in biliary colic results from distention of the biliary tree. Because the gallbladder muscle wall, and especially the muscle wall of the bile duct, is sparse, pain will occur that is severe and steady, as opposed to the pain of strong, intermittent contractions.

Most gallstones are composed primarily of cholesterol. Conditions that increase biliary secretion of cholesterol or decrease hepatic secretion of bile acids and phospholipids (e.g., obesity, rapid weight loss, aging) lead to supersaturation of bile with cholesterol, which can lead to the formation of cholesterol crystals and eventually stones. If gallbladder motility and emptying decreases (e.g., because of major surgery,

T ABLE 7.2. Risk factors for gallstone formation

CHOLESTEROL STONES
Female
Hispanic or Native American
Obesity (body mass index $\geq$30 kg/m^2)
Rapid weight loss
Pregnancy
Drugs [oral contraceptives, estrogens, clofibrate (Atromid-s); thiazides]
Age $\geq$50 years
Ileal disease or resection
Major surgery
Major burns
Total parenteral nutrition

CALCIUM BILIRUBINATE STONES
Chronic hemolytic states
Alcoholic cirrhosis
Chronic biliary tract infection

pregnancy, or use of total parenteral nutrition), biliary stasis can occur with the formation of biliary sludge. Biliary sludge is a thick mucous material containing cholesterol crystals, calcium bilirubinate, and mucin thread or mucous gels. Sludge is thought to be a precursor to gallstone formation. Cholesterol can play a role in sludge formation as studies show that excessive incorporation of cholesterol into the membranes of gallbladder smooth muscle cells causes gallbladder muscle dysfunction. The role of a genetic component in the development of gallstones is suggested by the identification of Lith 1 as a gallstone gene in inbred mice. In humans, the ApoE4 genotype is linked with increased intestinal absorption of cholesterol and the development of gallstones.

Gallstones can also be largely composed of calcium bilirubinate. These so-called pigment stones are seen in association with a chronic hemolytic state, alcoholic cirrhosis, and chronic biliary tract infection.

DIFFERENTIAL DIAGNOSIS

Causes of severe pain arising or chiefly localized to the right upper quadrant of the abdomen are listed in Table 7.3. Biliary colic generally can be distinguished from other biliary abnormalities by the presence of gallstones without additional abnormalities such as fever and an elevated WBC count (as would be seen in acute cholecystitis); fever, an elevated WBC count, markedly elevated alkaline phosphatase and bilirubin, and a dilated CBD (as would be seen in patients with cholangitis); fever, an elevated WBC count, abnormal liver function tests, dilated CBD, and elevated amylase (as would be seen in gallstone pancreatitis).

T ABLE 7.3.   Differential diagnosis of right upper quadrant pain

BILIARY CAUSES

Acute cholecystitis
Chronic cholecystitis
Cholangitis
Gallstone pancreatitis
Acalculous cholecystitis
Gallbladder cancer
Torsion of the gallbladder
Rupture of the gallbladder or cystic duct

NONBILIARY CAUSES

Peptic ulcer disease
Irritable bowel disease
Hepatitis
Pancreatitis
Coronary artery disease
Appendicitis
Renal pain or colic
Pleurisy
Pneumonia

If gallstones are not found, it is appropriate to look for other conditions such as peptic ulcer disease, irritable bowel syndrome, or hepatitis. However, in patients with a history highly suggestive of biliary colic but no stones seen on ultrasound, an HIDA scan can help diagnose acalculous cholecystitis.

Because asymptomatic gallstones are so common, taking a careful history should help the physician distinguish patients with nonbiliary causes of pain and silent gallstones from patients whose symptoms are caused by the gallstones.

REFERRAL

Patients with confirmed recurrent biliary colic generally should be referred for surgical consultation. A patient with evidence of acute cholecystitis should be hospitalized for evaluation, surgical consultation, and supportive measures. Consultation with a gastroenterologist may be needed for those patients who are unable to undergo surgery or who have symptoms of CBD obstruction.

MANAGEMENT

Patients with asymptomatic stones can expect a 2% to 3% chance of future biliary pain each year and less than 1% chance of presenting with a complication of biliary colic. Because of these low percentages, patients with asymptomatic gallstones generally do not need treatment.

Of patients who experience **a single episode of biliary colic**, 30% will experience no further pain or complications, 50% will have recurrent pain within 1 year, and 2% will experience a complication each year. Patients with a single episode of biliary colic are candidates for elective cholecystectomy but may choose watchful waiting to see if their pain reoccurs and should be supported if this is their decision. Restricting fat or cholesterol in the diet is of no proven benefit, but weight reduction through modest calorie restriction may be beneficial. Patients should be advised against taking estrogens, clofibrate (Atromid-S), and thiazides.

For patients with **recurrent biliary colic** and documented gallstones, **elective cholecystectomy** is recommended. Laparoscopic cholecystectomy, which became available in 1989, is now the most commonly performed elective abdominal surgery in the United States and the most common treatment for symptomatic gallstones. Laparoscopic cholecystectomy significantly shortens the patient's recovery time, compared with open cholecystectomy. Hospital stays for laparoscopic cholecystectomy are generally 1 to 2 days (with some centers studying same-day surgery options). Laparoscopic removal allows the patient to resume work in 3 to 10 days. Conversion to an open cholecystectomy is needed in approximately 5% of cases, usually because of poor visualization of the gallbladder.

Most patients with **acute cholecystitis** require **urgent cholecystectomy**. Morbidity and mortality rates are approximately fourfold higher for urgent surgery compared with elective surgery. Laparoscopic cholecystectomy is appropriate for many patients requiring urgent surgery, including elderly or pregnant patients.

For patients who either refuse surgery or who are poor candidates for elective surgery, consider **nonsurgical treatments**. Results from an oral cholecystogram can determine the most appropriate nonsurgical therapy. Patients in whom an oral cholecystogram shows a functioning gallbladder and small (<2 cm) radiolucent (i.e., cholesterol) stones can be placed on **oral bile acid therapy** [ursodiol (URSO)], at a dosage of 8 to 10 mg/kg/d given in two or three divided doses. Daily medication is continued for at least 12 months and often for 2 years. Oral bile acids act to dissolve cholesterol stones by increasing the solubility of cholesterol in the bile. The overall dissolution rate in a 2-year period is just under 50%, and 67% for "floating stones" (small, pure cholesterol stones that float during oral cholecystogram). Gallbladder ultrasound every 6 months is helpful in monitoring the success of therapy. Serum liver enzymes and cholesterol studies should be periodically obtained. Many patients become pain-free even before complete stone dissolution occurs. Oral bile acids are contraindicated in patients with inflammatory bowel disease or peptic ulcer disease because bile acids can be harmful to colonic and gastric mucosa. Fewer than 30% of patients with gallstones are candidates for oral bile acid therapy.

Another nonsurgical treatment for cholesterol stones is **topical dissolution** with methyl tert-butyl ether. This agent, which is repeatedly instilled into the gallbladder, dissolves cholesterol stones. An interventional radiologist passes a catheter percutaneously through the liver into the gallbladder. Stones of any size or number can be successfully treated with ether. The dissolution is rapid; however, topical dissolution is investigational and currently conducted in only a few centers. Complications can occur if the ether escapes into the peritoneal cavity or into the small intestine.

Extracorporeal shock wave lithotripsy uses acoustic shock waves to break stones into small pieces. After additional bile acid dissolution therapy, the small pieces may dissolve or pass into the small intestine. Stones should have a combined or additive diameter no greater than 3 cm. Lithotripsy with oral bile acid therapy in persons with a solitary 2-cm stone has a success rate of 60% within 6 months and 90% within 1 year. The procedure is contraindicated in patients with acute cholecystitis or a coagulation defect. Its availability has been limited by very high equipment costs, and its use has largely been supplanted by laparoscopic surgery. It remains a treatment option for patients with calcium-containing stones who are not surgical candidates.

Recurrence following all nonsurgical approaches is approximately 10% of patients each year for 5 years after initial dissolution. Recurrence is more common in patients who have multiple stones. Nonsurgical therapies, as opposed to cholecystectomy, do not prevent gallbladder cancer.

FOLLOW-UP

Potential Problems and Complications

Acute cholecystitis is acute inflammation of the gallbladder wall following obstruction of the cystic duct by a stone. It often begins as an attack of biliary colic that progressively worsens. Characteristically, the triad of sudden onset of RUQ tenderness, fever, and leukocytosis occurs. Murphy's sign (inspiratory arrest elicited when palpating the RUQ while asking the patient to take a deep breath) is often present. Serum transaminases and bilirubin may be mildly elevated. Ultrasound will demonstrate stones in 90% to 95% of cases. HIDA scan may be helpful in patients in whom the diagnosis of acute cholecystitis is in doubt. Surgical consultation is warranted at first suspicion as acute cholecystitis is best treated with early cholecystectomy. Seriously ill or debilitated patients can be managed with cholecystostomy and tube drainage with elective cholecystectomy done at a later time.

Acalculous cholecystitis refers to the 5% to 10% of patients with acute cholecystitis with no stones found on imaging or at surgery. In more than 50% of such cases an underlying explanation for gallbladder inflammation is not found. An increased risk for developing acalculous cholecystitis exists in patients with severe trauma or burns, in the postpartum period, or following major surgery. Other precipitating factors include: vasculitis; adenocarcinoma of the gallbladder; unusual bacterial or parasitic infections of the gallbladder; and with other systemic processes (e.g., sarcoidosis, tuberculosis), or with prolonged parenteral hyperalimentation. HIDA scan is useful for diagnosis.

Acalculous cholecystopathy is disordered motility of the gallbladder that produces recurrent biliary pain in patients without stones. It is diagnosed by an infusion of cholecystokinin during an HIDA scan. Diagnostic criteria include a low (< 40%) ejection fraction and the cholecystokinin infusion reproducing the patient's pain.

Emphysematous cholecystitis is acute cholecystitis followed by ischemia or gangrene of the gallbladder wall and infection by gas-producing organisms. This condition occurs most frequently in elderly men and diabetics. Diagnosis is made by finding gas within the gallbladder lumen or wall on plain abdominal films. Prompt surgical intervention coupled with appropriate antibiotics is mandatory as morbidity and mortality are considerable with this condition.

Chronic cholecystitis is chronic inflammation of the gallbladder wall. It is almost always associated with the presence of gallstones and is thought to be the result of repeated bouts of subacute or acute cholecystitis or from persistent mechanical irritation of the gallbladder wall from increased intraluminal pressures and distention. Chronic cholecystitis can be asymptomatic for years or progress to symptomatic gallbladder disease, to acute cholecystitis, or to other complications of stone disease.

Complications of cholecystectomy include atelectasis, abscess formation, hemorrhage, biliary-enteric fistula, and bile leaks. Routine performance of intraoperative choliangiography during cholecystectomy has helped to reduce the incidence of biliary tract complications. The overall complication rate for laparoscopic cholecystectomy is similar to open cholecystectomy (5%), but serious complications, which include bile duct injuries with bile leaks and stricture formation, occur two to three times more frequently with laparoscopic surgery (0.5% vs. 0.2%). Mortality rates are similar for laparoscopic and open cholecystectomy: less than 0.1% for elective surgery and approximately 3% for urgent surgery (higher if significant underlying illnesses are present). Bile duct injuries can result in considerable patient disability.

Postcholecystectomy syndrome refers to the persistence of symptoms after surgical removal of the gallbladder. It occurs in approximately 4% of cholecystectomy patients. The most common cause is an overlooked extrabiliary disorder (e.g., reflux esophagitis, peptic ulceration, pancreatitis, or irritable bowel syndrome) as the cause of the patient's symptoms. A small percent, however, will have the postcholecystectomy syndrome caused by (a) biliary strictures, (b) retained biliary stone in the common bile duct, (c) cystic duct stump syndrome, (d) stenosis or dyskinesia of the Oddi's sphincter, or (e) bile salt-induced diarrhea or gastritis.

Cholangitis is a complication of stones in the common bile duct (choledocholithiasis) causing obstruction to bile flow and infection. Acute cholangitis presents with Charcot's triad: biliary colic, jaundice, and spiking fevers with chills. Elevated WBC count, hyperbilirubinemia, elevated alkaline phosphatase, and positive blood cultures are expected. Broad spectrum antibiotics (which provide coverage against gram-positive enterococci, gram-negative enterobacter, and anaerobes) and endoscopic retrograde cholangiopancreatography with endoscopic sphincterotomy is the preferred initial procedure for both establishing a definitive diagnosis and providing effective treatment. It can be difficult to distinguish acute cholecystitis from cholangitis. Ultrasound will diagnose gallbladder stones and common bile duct size but is poor at demonstrating CBD stones. If cholangitis is suspected, preoperative choliangiography may be necessary.

Gallstone pancreatitis occurs when a gallstone becomes lodged in the CBD and obstructs the pancreatic duct. Pancreatic inflammation with elevated amylase values is seen in approximately 15% of acute cholecystitis cases and in more than 30% of choledocholithiasis patients. In addition to typical symptoms of acute cholecystitis, back pain or left abdominal pain, prolonged vomiting with paralytic ileus, or a left-sided pleural effusion would commonly be seen. Diagnosis is usually made by cholangiography and treated by endoscopic sphincterotomy and stone extraction by endoscopic retrograde cholangiopancreatography.

Gallbladder cancer is associated with gallstone disease. The incidence is higher in persons with symptomatic stones than asymptomatic. Although increased, the risk is still low (0.02% cases/year). Prophylactic cholecystectomy has only been considered for high risk groups like the Pima Indians or those with a porcelain gallbladder (patients with a chronically inflamed gallbladder and calcium salt deposition within the gallbladder wall detectable by plain abdominal films).

PATIENT EDUCATION

Patients with asymptomatic stones are at low risk of future gallstone problems and need no further treatment or follow-up unless biliary colic occurs. Restricting fat or cholesterol in the diet is of no proven benefit, but weight reduction through modest calorie restriction may be beneficial to these patients. These patients should probably be advised against taking estrogens, clofibrate, and thiazides.

Patients with a single episode of biliary colic can be counseled similarly. However, with a much higher rate of recurrent pain likely, some patients may prefer a surgical consultation to prevent further episodes of pain.

Patients with recurrent biliary colic or with a history of a gallstone complication warrant surgical consultation. Patients can be informed of the advantages (quicker recovery times) and disadvantages (increased risk of serious bile leak complications) of laparoscopic surgery.

For those patients unwilling or unable to undergo surgery, an oral cholecystogram should be performed to help guide the selection of nonsurgical treatments. Primarily calcified stones would be candidates for lithotripsy; cholesterol stones are candidates for oral bile acid therapy.

Patients with known gallstones can confuse dyspepsia with biliary colic. The distinction between the two should be emphasized and should make clear that gallstone treatment will not alleviate the dyspepsia.

SUGGESTED READING

Cope's early diagnosis of the acute abdomen, 17th ed, rev. Silen W ed. Oxford University Press, 1987:115-116, 129-130, 147-150.

Goroll AH, May LA, Mulley AG. Jr., eds. Management of asymptomatic and symptomatic gallstones. In: *Primary care medicine: office evaluation and management of the adult patient*, 3rd ed. Philadelphia: Lippincott Williams & Wilkins; 1995:394-399.

Howard D, Fromm H. Nonsurgical management of gallstone disease. *Gastroenterol Clin North Am* 1999;28(1):133-144.

Greenberger NJ, Isselbacher KJ. Diseases of the gallbladder and bile ducts. In: Fauci *Harrison's principles of internal medicine*, 14th ed. New York: McGraw Hill; 1998:1726-1733.

Ransohoff D, Gracie W. Treatment of gallstones. *Ann Intern Med* 1993;119(7): 606-619.

CHAPTER 8

Dysphagia

Kurt Kurowski

DEFINITION

Dysphagia is defined as the impairment or the sensation of impairment of swallowing. It is traditionally divided into oropharyngeal dysphagia and esophageal dysphagia. Disorders occurring in the first phase of swallowing relating to the mouth and pharynx result in oropharyngeal dysphagia; those occurring later more typically result in esophageal dysphagia. Individuals with esophageal dysphagia may complain of food sticking behind the sternum or the need to consciously swallow, perhaps several times, for food to pass down.

PATIENT HISTORY

Associated symptoms are sometimes the predominant or even the only symptoms of many of the disorders that can produce dysphagia.

Odynophagia, or painful swallowing, is associated with oropharyngeal inflammation, pill-induced esophagitis, caustic chemical ingestion, infection, or carcinoma. Among esophageal infections, herpes simplex usually causes more odynophagia and less dysphagia, whereas *Candida* or cytomegalovirus infection can produce either symptom or both.

Coughing from aspiration or dyspnea after eating is a frequent manifestation of oropharyngeal dysphagia. It can also be seen with esophageal dysphagia if backlogged food rises to the epiglottis. The patient may also experience reflux symptoms, including a sensation of acidic material ascending into the oropharynx, especially with recumbency. Depending on the specific disorder responsible, chest pains can be experienced during or after eating, or without any particular prandial association.

Aggravating or Alleviating Factors and Symptom Progression

Food consistency. Patients with oropharyngeal dysphagia will usually aspirate less with puréed foods. They tend to have more difficulty with liquids than with solids.

Esophageal dysphagia that begins with chewy foods (e.g., steaks and bread), then progresses to include other solid foods, and, eventually, to liquids suggests an obstruction. A benign mechanical obstruction (e.g., a peptic stricture or esophageal ring) is likely if this progression took years to develop. Esophageal carcinoma is more likely if the progression occurs over weeks to months. Intermittent esophageal dysphagia for both liquids and solids suggests an esophageal motility disorder.

Other Historical Clues for Specific Causes

Weight loss typically suggests esophageal carcinoma but can be seen in association with esophagitis secondary to *Candida* or herpes simplex virus.

TABLE 8.1. Medications associated with dysphagia

Via direct inflammatory response in esophagus	Via aggravation of gastroesophageal reflux	Via aggravation of xerostomia
Alendronate sodium (Fosamax)	Calcium channel blockers	Antispasmodics
Potassium chloride (Slow-K)	Nitrates	Antidepressants[a]
Tetracycline or doxycycline (Vibramycin)	Theophylline	Antihistamines
Ferrous sulfate or succinate	Progesterone	Antiparkinson agents[b]
Aspirin	Anticholinergics	Antipsychotics
Vitamin C	Alpha blockers or beta agonists	
Quinidine	Sedatives	
Phenytoin (Dilantin)		
Theophylline (slow release)		
Clindamycin (Cleocin)		

[a]Includes tricyclic antidepressants and selective serotonin reuptake inhibitors (SSRIS).
[b]Includes anticholinergic, dopaminergic and catechol O-methyltransferase inhibitors.

Fever. The combination of fever and dysphagia is usually secondary to aspiration pneumonia caused by oropharyngeal dysphagia. Malignancy, esophagitis, or pharyngitis can also cause fever.

Skin changes. Tightening of the skin or Raynaud's phenomenon suggests esophageal dysmotility secondary to progressive systemic sclerosis.

Oral lesions. Patients with esophageal candidiasis usually have oral thrush, particularly those with the acquired immune deficiency syndrome. A minority of patients with herpes simplex esophagitis will have concomitant oral or cutaneous herpes. A dry mouth, especially in an elderly patient who has had radiation treatments to the head and neck or is receiving possible exacerbating medications (Table 8.1), suggests xerostomia.

Human immunodeficiency virus (HIV) infection or other immunocompromised states. Esophagitis secondary to *Candida*, herpes simplex virus, or cytomegalovirus is almost entirely confined to these groups.

Neurologic disease. Stroke is the most common cause of oropharyngeal dysphagia. Dysphagia can also be a manifestation of transient ischemic attacks. Patients with Alzheimer's disease and Parkinson's disease frequently experience oropharyngeal dysphagia. Dysphagia seen with spastic paresis combined with fasciculations and atrophy suggests amyotrophic lateral sclerosis. Fatigable weakness in primarily bulbar musculature suggests myasthenia gravis.

Other gastrointestinal complaints. Symptoms of reflux that began before dysphagia symptoms suggest reflux esophagitis or peptic stricture. Regurgitation of previously ingested food suggests a Zenker's diverticulum, which is a pouch opening into the hypopharynx.

Ingestions or Exposures Suggesting Specific Causes of Dysphagia

Caustic ingestion. Lye (e.g., potassium hydroxide), ammonium, or various acids will produce immediate necrosis. Scarring of the esophagus begins 1 week after exposure and progresses over 3 months. Table 8.2 lists the trade names and chemical components of the caustic agents most commonly found in patients' households.

T ABLE 8.2. Caustic agents

Chemical agent	Commercial products
Acids	
Acetic acid	Permanent wave neutralizers
Boric acid	Water softeners
Cantharides (Spanish fly)	Aphrodisiacs, hair ionics, abortifacients
Formaldehyde (formic acid)	Deodorizing tablets, plastic menders, fumigants, embalming agents
Hydrochloric (muriatic) acid, sulfuric acid	Metal and toilet bowl cleaners
Hydrofluoric acid, sulfuric acid	Antirust products
Oxalic acid	Disinfectants, household bleach, metal cleaning fluids, antirust products, furniture polish
Phenol (creosol)	Antiseptics, preservatives
Phosphoric acid, sulfuric acid	Toilet bowl cleaners
Alkalis	
Sodium hydroxide	
96%–100%	Red Devil Drain Opener
50%	Crystalline Drano
2%–10%	Liquid Drano
Sodium carbonate	Mr. Clean Liquid
Sodium carbonate plus ammonia	Top Job Liquid
Sodium hypochlorite (5.25%)	Liquid Clorox
Ammonium chloride	
2.7%	Lysol Deodorizing Cleaner
1.25%	Swish Toilet Bowl Cleaner
Miscellaneous	
Manganese dioxide, lithium, mercuric oxide, nickel-cadmium, silver oxide, zinc-air	Disk batteries
Iodine	Antiseptics
Phosphorus	Matches, rodenticides, insecticides, fireworks
Potassium permanganate	Abortifacients, topical medicines

Reprinted from Spiegelman GA, Rogers AI. Chemical injury of the esophagus. In: Haubrich WS, Schaffner F, Berk JE, eds. *Gastroenterology*, 5th ed. Philadelphia: WB Saunders, 1995:483–489; with permission.

Medications. Pills that disintegrate within the esophagus can produce local inflammation and symptoms. Commonly implicated medications are alendronate (Fosamax), doxycycline (Vibramycin), potassium chloride tablets (Slow-K), iron tablets, and nonsteroidal antiinflammatory drugs. Other medications can cause dysphagia by producing or aggravating gastrointestinal reflux or xerostomia. Table 8.1 lists medications associated with dysphagia. Pill-induced strictures can occur at the distal esophagus, especially with alendronate (Fosamax), but more often occur at the level of the aortic arch. Strictures are more likely in elderly patients and in cases of some obstruction or decreased motility of the esophagus. Taking medications with at least 120 ml of water diminishes the likelihood of pills lodging in the esophagus.

Radiation. Strictures or motility problems of the esophagus can develop months to years after mediastinal radiation. These complications are unusual for radiation exposures of less than 30 Gy.

PHYSICAL EXAMINATION

The physical examination is limited in the evaluation of a patient with dysphagia because of the inaccessibility of the esophagus to examination.

Oropharynx. Careful inspection for inflammation, swelling, ulcers, or tumors that might interfere with food chewing and swallowing may identify the problem. Poor dentition or ill-fitting dentures are common contributors to a solid food oropharyngeal dysphagia that is seen, especially in the elderly. Observation of the patient swallowing both solids and liquids is useful for assessing aspiration and oropharyngeal dysphagia.

Neck. Cervical adenopathy can be an indicator of inflammation or malignancy within the oropharynx. Thyroid enlargement that could be compressing the proximal esophagus may be detected on examination. Palpation of an esophageal diverticulum can cause expression of its contents into the esophagus and oropharynx.

Supraclavicular fossa. Mediastinal infection or malignancy, including those compressing or originating from the esophagus, can produce supraclavicular adenopathy.

Lungs. Crackles and rhonchi can develop (usually in the dependent segments of the lung) from aspiration secondary to oropharyngeal dysphagia or from regurgitation from esophageal obstruction. The patient can often clear these sounds with coughing. Consolidation signs are usually absent even with aspiration pneumonia.

Abdomen. The esophageal transit time estimation test may help in the examination. The patient can be instructed to drink a glass of water while the examiner listens via a stethoscope over the left upper quadrant for the sound of the water entering the stomach while timing the interval from the swallow. A normal transit time is 7 to 10 seconds; a delay suggests intrinsic or extrinsic obstruction.

Neurologic examination. Motor and sensory examinations, cranial nerve testing, deep tendon reflexes, and gait assessment are all appropriate because neurologic disorders and myopathies can produce oropharyngeal dysphagia as a prominent and sometimes first manifestation.

DIAGNOSTIC STUDIES

Initial workup for oropharyngeal dysphagia includes a video swallowing study and usually a clinical evaluation of swallowing by a speech therapist. Typically, a speech therapist observes the ingestion of liquid, puréed, and solid materials to detect defects in the swallowing mechanism and assess the risk for aspiration. An esophagram (barium swallow) is considered if the video-swallowing study is normal. In suspected esophageal dysphagia, the workup begins with either an esophagram or endoscopy. The latter is preferred in cases where structural lesions or esophagitis are suspected.

If yeast infection is suspected, brushings from endoscopy samples can be mounted on a slide with a 10% potassium hydroxide solution and examined for yeast cells and pseudohyphae to confirm candidiasis. Fungal cultures of biopsy material can also be obtained. Inclusion bodies will be seen in ulcer sites of herpetic and cytomegalovirus esophagitis. Immunocytologic studies and specific viral cultures can identify cytomegalovirus or herpes simplex. **Stool guaiac** examination may be posi-

T ABLE 8.3. Appropriate use of blood tests in the evaluation of dysphagia

Disease (suspected)	Blood study
Esophagitis	Some cases will have leukocytosis
Myositis	Creatinine phosphokinase elevation
Diabetes mellitus	Fasting serum glucose
Electrolyte imbalance	Serum electrolyte abnormality
Hypothyroidism	Thyroid-stimulating hormone
Myasthenia gravis	AchR (anticholinesterase receptor) antibodies
Wilson's disease	Ceruloplasmin level
Systemic sclerosis	Antinuclear antibodies with a nucleolar pattern (Anti Scl-70 or anticentromere antibodies are more specific)
Recurrent squamous cell carcinoma of esophagus	CA 19-9 (not sensitive enough for screening or initial diagnosis)
Botulism	Botulinum toxin (from serum and stool)

tive in cases of esophageal malignancy or esophagitis. **Blood tests** typically provide little help in the evaluation. Exceptions to this general rule are presented in Table 8.3.

Esophageal manometry is used only in cases of suspected achalasia or esophageal motility disorders. A 24-hour manometry with software analysis provides excellent characterization and classification of esophageal motor events.

RISK FACTORS

Squamous cell carcinoma of the esophagus is much more likely in individuals who have a history of tobacco use in any form (i.e., cigarettes, cigars, pipes, and smokeless tobacco) and in those with chronic alcohol abuse (especially of distilled liquors). Alcohol and tobacco consumption together produce a dramatic synergistic increase in risk. Squamous cell esophageal carcinoma is more common in African-American patients than in white patients. Patients with Plummer-Vinson syndrome (spoon-shaped nails, esophageal web, angular stomatitis), tylosis (autosomal-dominant hyperkeratosis of palms and soles), or those who have had partial gastrectomy are at increased risk. An association appears to exist between human papillomavirus (HPV) and esophageal dysplasia and squamous cell carcinoma. Also, multiple potential environmental and dietary risk factors exist, including the drinking of certain herbal teas served at very hot temperatures that are popular in some Latin American cultures.

Adenocarcinoma of the esophagus is usually secondary to malignant transformation of a Barrett's esophagus (see Chapter 9). Approximately 10% to 15% of patients who develop a Barrett's esophagus will later develop adenocarcinoma. Gastroesophageal reflux (especially if it is severe) is a risk factor for adenocarcinoma of the esophagus, even if transformation to Barrett's esophagus does not occur.

Peptic strictures are sequelae of persistent gastroesophageal reflux. Esophageal motility disorders and Schatzki's rings are also associated with reflux.

Pill-induced strictures are more likely in cases of preexistent obstruction or a motility disorder in the esophagus.

EPIDEMIOLOGY

The epidemiology of dysphagia depends on its cause. Overall, more dysphagia is seen in the elderly with other medical problems. It is estimated that 12% of patients during acute hospital stays and 60% of nursing home patients experience dysphagia.

PATHOPHYSIOLOGY

Swallowing involves the coordination of several neuromuscular events. Food is initially chewed and mixed with saliva; the tongue then forms a bolus against the palate. With the voluntary start of the swallow, the mouth and jaw close and the anterior tongue touches the hard palate while the middle and posterior portions push the bolus into the oropharynx. The pharynx then involuntarily develops peristalsis, and the soft palate elevates as the larynx elevates and moves anteriorly, closing the epiglottis, thus protecting the airway. Neurologic or muscular disorders affecting the multiple cranial nerves involved in these processes, or of the brainstem swallowing center, can result in oropharyngeal dysphagia. A lack of adequate saliva production will also cause this through inadequate bolus lubrication. Any obstructive lesion or diverticulum along the tract can also produce this type of dysphagia.

The esophageal phase begins with the involuntary opening of the upper esophageal sphincter followed by a wave of coordinated peristalsis down the body of the esophagus with the lower esophageal sphincter opening as the bolus reaches the distal esophagus. Obstructive lesions within the esophagus, including mucosa inflammation, will produce esophageal dysphagia. Abnormalities of the muscular peristaltic wave or in sphincter relaxation, as in the esophageal motility disorders, will also produce this symptom.

DIFFERENTIAL DIAGNOSIS

Once the patient is identified as having dysphagia, the first step is to differentiate between oropharyngeal and esophageal dysphagia. This is important because the potential causes, diagnostic evaluations, and treatment differ greatly. However, because food and liquid can sometimes backlog into the oropharynx and produce oropharyngeal symptoms from esophageal dysphagia, differentiation on symptoms alone is often not possible. Figure 8.1 is an algorithm that summarizes the key issues in the diagnostic approach.

Oropharyngeal dysphagia is suggested when the patient complains of a sense of food sticking in, or not clearing from, the throat. Coughing, especially after eating, can be another indicator, as is hoarseness. The patient may have difficulty initiating a swallow and experience aspiration. Table 8.4 presents common causes for oropharyngeal dysphagia.

Esophageal dysphagia is sensed after swallowing has been completed. No sense of, or evidence for, aspiration occurs if there is no backlog into the oropharynx. A sense should be felt that liquid and food are not passing at their normal rates from the proximal esophagus into the stomach and the patient may experience substernal chest pain. Most patients with esophageal obstructions (74%) can accurately identify the level of their lesion. Table 8.5 presents common causes for esophageal dysphagia.

Although clues from the history sometimes provide a ready diagnosis (i.e., pharyngitis, pill-induced dysphagia), they are more likely to suggest only an oropharyngeal or esophageal source and possibly an obstructing lesion. Imaging or endoscopic evaluation is usually necessary to reach a diagnosis.

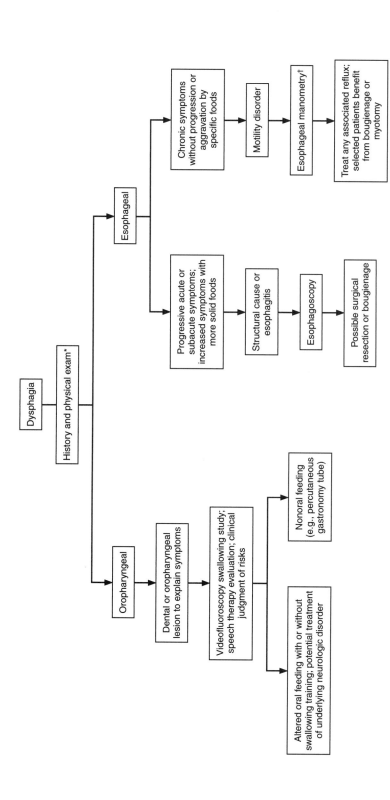

FIGURE 8.1. Algorithm for diagnosis and causes of dysphagia.

*Differentiating between oropharyngeal and esophageal dysphagia is not always possible on history and physical examination. Evaluate for the other type of dysphagia if work-up of initially suspected source is negative.

†Associated gastroesophageal reflux and infiltrating carcinoma may mimic or exacerbate motility disorders. Esophagoscopy and pH monitoring are therefore usually used in the initial evaluation.

T ABLE 8.4. Differential diagnosis for oropharyngeal dysphagia

COMMON NEUROLOGIC CAUSES[a]
Cerebrovascular accident or transient ischemia of hemispheres or brain stem
Central nervous system trauma (including surgical) or neoplasm
Amyotrophic lateral sclerosis (oropharyngeal dysphagia is a common first presentation)
Multiple sclerosis
Cranial nerve disease (especially of recurrent laryngeal nerve)
Parkinson's disease
Myasthenia gravis
Alzheimer's disease

COMMON MUSCULAR CAUSES
Dermatomyositis or polymyositis
Myotonic dystrophy
Sarcoidosis

LOCAL INFLAMMATION OR OBSTRUCTION
Pharyngitis
Zenker's diverticulum
Cricopharyngeal bar or web
Oropharyngeal malignancy
Compression secondary to thyromegaly, cervical spine spurs or lymphadenopathy

POOR FOOD BOLUS FORMATION
Xerostomia
Poor denture fit or dental problems

[a]Less common causes include botulism, Lyme disease, syphilis, polio, Guillain-Barré syndrome, Wilson's disease, and Huntington's disease.

T ABLE 8.5. Differential diagnosis for esophageal dysphagia

STRUCTURAL LESIONS	EXTERNAL COMPRESSION
STRICTURES	**FUNCTIONAL ABNORMALITIES**
Peptic (or gastroesophageal reflux-associated) stricture	Gastroesophageal reflux disease without stricture
Scarring from caustic ingestion or radiation	Achalasia
Pill-induced	Diffuse esophageal spasm
	Nutcracker esophagus
CARCINOMA OF ESOPHAGUS	Hypertensive lower esophageal sphincter
	Chagas' disease
ESOPHAGITIS	Metabolic esophageal motor abnormalities
Infectious	Diabetes mellitus
Acute or subacute caustic or radiation injury	Hypothyroidism
Pill-induced injury	Electrolyte abnormalities
	Medication-induced
SCHATZKI'S RING OR WEBS	Progressive systemic sclerosis

REFERRAL

Most cases of oropharyngeal dysphagia presenting to the family physician involve already recognized neurologic disease (e.g., stroke, Alzheimer's disease). In such cases, definitive management by the family physician is usually possible with the assistance of a speech therapist.

Table 8.6 presents dietary recommendations for some of the more commonly encountered causes of dysphagia. Dialogue between dietitians and speech therapists allows more individualized recommendations, including those for other types of dysphagia not listed in this table. Neurologic consultation is appropriate if the neurologic cause of the dysphagia cannot be identified. Gastroenterologic consultation may also be helpful where the cause of the dysphagia still cannot be identified or when the response to therapy is judged to be inadequate. Surgical or gastrointestinal consultation is warranted if a gastrostomy tube is being considered or if obstructive causes have been identified.

Most patients with esophageal dysphagia require an endoscopic evaluation of the esophagus and, thus, would be referred to either a gastroenterologist or a general surgeon early in the course of their evaluation. Physicians in either one of these specialties usually have experience with dilatation procedures in the esophagus, if necessary. The decreased morbidity of laparoscopic and thoracoscopic techniques compared with older procedures will increase the use of fundoplication procedures for reflux and surgical myotomy in the treatment of achalasia.

MANAGEMENT

Management depends on the specific diagnosis. Oral feeding should be withheld or thicker food substances used in the management of oropharyngeal dysphagia pending evaluation.

T ABLE 8.6.   Dietary recommendations for selected causes of dysphagia

Cause	Dietary recommendations
Xerostomia	Ensure adequate liquid intake and consider use of artificial saliva. Moist, well-lubricated foods are best; add gravies, sauces, and butter to accomplish this. Avoid foods that crumble apart (e.g., plain rice, whole-grain breads, ground meats).
Poor swallowing reflex or reduced swallowing coordination secondary to stroke, Alzheimer's disease, Parkinson's disease, and so on	Cohesive foods (e.g., soft cheeses, meatloaf, casseroles, salads with mayonnaise) are best. A swallowing reflex may be better elicited with foods that are more seasoned or served closer to temperature extremes. Commercial thickeners should be added to any thin liquids.
Decreased esophageal peristalsis (e.g., achalasia, Chagas' disease)	Dense foods (e.g., meatloaf, mashed potatoes, lasagna) are best and may be followed by liquids. Foods with a sticky consistency (e.g., peanut butter) should be avoided.
Esophageal obstruction secondary to tumor, Schatzki's ring	Thin liquids (e.g., fruit juices, citrus juices, milk, broth, soda) are tolerated best followed by pureed or soft foods. Thick, chewy foods (e.g., steaks, breads) are poorly tolerated, as are sticky foods such as peanut butter.

Oropharyngeal dysphagia secondary to neurologic or muscular disease can sometimes be ameliorated with medication directed at the underlying disorder (e.g., Parkinson's disease, myasthenia gravis). Inflammatory myopathies are treated with corticosteroids, sometimes in combination with azathioprine (Imuran) or methotrexate. However, neither of these agents has US Food and Drug Administration (FDA) approval for this indication. Intravenous immunoglobulin is helpful for inclusion body myositis but does not have an FDA indication for this use. Even if treatment for the underlying disorder is not possible, swallowing training and thickening of liquids is often helpful (Tables 8.6 and 8.7). Debilitated, lethargic patients often have dramatic improvement in their oropharyngeal dysphagia with improvement in their general status. Many patients will continue to experience dysphagia and even aspiration despite these efforts, or are judged at the onset to be unlikely to improve adequately with the aforementioned measures. These patients require an alternative non-oral feeding method, usually placement of a percutaneous gastrostomy tube.

Oropharyngeal dysphagia secondary to obstruction sometimes requires surgical intervention. A smaller (< 5 cm in diameter) Zenker's diverticulum can be surgically suspended to the prevertebral fascia through a left cervical incision. Larger diverticula are excised. The radiographic identification of cricopharyngeal bars (an indentation in the region of the upper esophageal sphincter caused by a spastic cricopharyngeus muscle) must be judged with caution, as most of these bars do not produce dysphagia. Cricopharyngeal myotomy can relieve dysphagia in the few patients where this lesion is truly responsible, but manometry and esophagoscopy to search for other causes should be done first. Extrinsic compression from enlarged thyroids or cervical exostoses can be relieved by excision of the compressing components of these structures.

Esophageal dysphagia secondary to structural lesions can usually be at least temporarily improved with dilatation of the obstruction. Peptic stricture progression can be retarded with the use of a histamine$_2$ (H$_2$) receptor antagonist or a proton pump inhibitor in conjunction with mechanical efforts to reduce reflux. Proton pump inhibitors are considered more effective for this purpose as they also decrease

---

T ABLE 8.7. Aspiration-reducing feeding maneuvers for oropharyngeal dysphagia

SET-UP AND POSITIONING FOR FEEDING
Feeding should take place in an environment free of distractions
The patient should be fully upright with feet flat on floor
The patient's head is tilted slightly forward

PACE AND METHOD OF FEEDING
Encourage small bites
Encourage frequent dry swallows to clear mouth of food
Discourage use of liquids to clear mouth of food

CARETAKER SAFETY CHECKS
Periodically check voice quality between swallows (a gurgling voice could indicate that food is adjacent to vocal cords and has not been swallowed into esophagus)
Observe for rise in Adam's apple with each swallow (lack of rise could indicate food retention in mouth or pharynx)

the severity of esophagitis and the sensation of dysphagia in patients with peptic stricture, thus reducing the need for stricture dilatation.

If symptomatic strictures are present, bougienage (the passage of large-caliber dilators) can be effective, but usually has to be repeated when symptoms recur. Strictures secondary to a caustic injury are best prevented by stent placement in the subacute phase of the injury.

Schatzki's ring (lower esophageal ring) should be treated initially with reassurance and patient instruction in slow, meticulous mastication. Schatzki's ring is associated with gastroesophageal reflux. If identified, the reflux should be treated. In refractory cases, consider endoscopic electrosurgical disruption of the ring or surgical excision.

Surgical resection is usually attempted for **esophageal carcinoma**. Transthoracic esophagectomy with excision of periesophageal lymph nodes is the most common surgical approach, but transhiatal approaches are also used, especially for tumors of the lower third of the esophagus. Patients with stage I (tumor confined to submucosa) or stage II (tumor confined to muscularis layer or adventitia) lesions have a dramatically better prognosis with resection (60% 5-year survival with stage I and ~ 30% 5-year survival with stage II), but only about 10% of squamous cell carcinoma cases are diagnosed in these early stages. Endoscopic ultrasonography and computed tomography of the chest allow recognition of stage III (regional metastases or tumor invasion into adjacent structures) and stage IV (distant metastases) disease. Stage IV should be treated with palliation. Stage III has only a 10% to 20% 5-year survival rate after surgical resection. Adenocarcinoma of the esophagus also usually presents at advanced stages, and has similar surgical outcomes. However, patients undergoing surveillance endoscopies for Barrett's esophagus do fare better. These tumors are almost always in stage I or II when detected. Unfortunately, most cases of squamous cell carcinoma have local extension beyond the resection site, and many adenocarcinomas have distant metastases, making surgical cure unusual.

Palliative therapy for esophageal carcinoma. Dilatation procedures as described above for benign lesions are usually effective for palliation. Endoscopic laser therapy, fluoroscopic- or endoscopic-directed electrocoagulation, or esophageal stenting are also effective. Combining endoscopic laser therapy with intravenous photosensitizers in what is called "photodynamic therapy" may produce even better responses. Squamous cell carcinomas are more likely to respond to palliative radiation than are adenocarcinomas. Some centers combine intraluminal and external-beam radiation to minimize injury to periesophageal structures.

Esophageal dysphagia secondary to gastroesophageal reflux without stricture should initially be addressed with lifestyle modifications (e.g., losing weight if obese; elevating the head of the bed with a 6- to 8-inch Styrofoam wedge under the mattress; stopping smoking; decreasing fat intake; and avoiding recumbency after eating). Medications that could aggravate reflux should be reduced or discontinued if possible. H_2 receptor antagonists or prokinetic agents are prescribed. In more severe or persistent cases, proton pump inhibitors are prescribed for 4 weeks. These same symptom control strategies, especially the proton pump inhibitor, help reduce the chances of eventual stricture formation. Patients with associated incompetent lower esophageal sphincters, with particularly severe esophagitis secondary to reflux, at higher risk for adenocarcinoma, or with an incomplete response to medical therapy should be considered for antireflux surgery. It is also an option for good surgical risk candidates aged less than 60 years who do not wish to take chronic acid suppressant medications for the long term. Laparoscopic fundoplication will cure the dysphagia in approximately 90% of cases.

Esophageal dysphagia secondary to motility disorders is treated based on the specific disorder identified. **Achalasia** (a disease of unknown cause with a loss of myenteric neurons with resultant poor lower esophageal sphincter relaxation and esophageal peristalsis) is most commonly treated with pneumatic dilatation of the lower esophageal sphincter. Most patients with achalasia require only one dilatation and 70% to 80% respond to this treatment. Perforations sometimes occur (3% of patients), and many patients experience gastroesophageal reflux after the dilatation. Laparoscopic Heller's myotomy has an even higher response rate (80% to 90%), but is even more likely to produce reflux. Most surgeons perform an antireflux procedure along with the myotomy to reduce this risk. Botulinum toxin type A injection into the lower esophageal sphincter is also usually successful (but not FDA approved for this indication) and has a lower complication rate, but patients require costly repeat injections. Its use is usually limited to patients who are poor risks for, or are unwilling to accept the risks of, definitive surgical treatment. The myenteric neurons can also be destroyed by *Trypanosoma cruzi* in **Chagas' disease**, which is endemic to South America. Esophageal symptoms develop many years after the acute infection. The symptoms are the same as those of achalasia and the esophageal manifestations are treated the same way.

Other motility disorders of the esophagus, including diffuse and segmental esophageal spasms, the nutcracker esophagus, and nonspecific esophageal motility disorder, have similar treatment. Some of these disorders are seen in the same patients on manometry studies taken at different times, suggesting that they may not be distinct from each other. Most of these patients also have reflux. An aggressive search for and treatment of reflux is warranted, particularly when the chief complaint is chest pain, because the reflux may be producing spasm. Dilatation and bougienage have been successful in some patients with spastic disorders of the esophagus. A long esophageal myotomy can be beneficial to some patients, but it should only be considered when the chief complaint is dysphagia, not chest pain.

FOLLOW-UP

Although patients complaining of dysphagia initially merit a fairly extensive evaluation as described above, most do not require reevaluation if their symptoms remain under control with therapy. Several exceptions are found, however. If lower esophageal biopsies reveal Barrett's esophagus (metaplasia of the squamous epithelium into columnar epithelium), repeat endoscopies and biopsies are warranted because some patients will develop adenocarcinoma of the esophagus, even if they are asymptomatic. Definitive surveillance timing has not been established, but most centers recommend annual endoscopy if biopsies and cytology are negative for dysplasia. Flow cytometry analysis can also be used to detect aneuploidy or increased tetraploid fractions, which correlate with dysplasia. If biopsies and cytology show no dysplasia and flow cytometry is negative, surveillance endoscopies can be repeated in 2 years. Many patients treated with dilatation of the esophagus or bougienage will require retreatment, especially if they are followed over a course of 5 years. The need for retreatment and the increased risk for carcinoma, even in patients with benign strictures, suggest that these patients should have repeat endoscopies with the capacity to perform repeat dilatation if symptoms recur.

PATIENT EDUCATION

Patients with **oropharyngeal dysphagia** or with conditions that place them at risk for its development and their family and caretakers need to be aware of the symptoms. Difficulties initiating or completing a swallow or the development of a cough after eating can indicate this type of dysphagia and resultant aspiration. Many patients with oropharyngeal dysphagia have undergone swallowing training, and it is useful if family and caretakers are aware of the need for the patient to be in a fully upright position during feeding, as well as the appropriate speed of feeding and allowable food consistencies (Table 8.6). Helpful maneuvers during swallowing (e.g., head tilts) should be understood by caretakers so they can see that the maneuvers are being used at each feeding (Table 8.7).

The most critical issue for a patient with esophageal dysphagia is to recognize that any new onset dysphagia or progression of dysphagia (e.g., softer foods begin to produce dysphagia) could represent esophageal carcinoma. Early assessment is crucial. Known risk behaviors for esophageal carcinoma (e.g., tobacco and alcohol use) should be discouraged.

SUGGESTED READING

Alrakawi A, Clouse RE. The changing use of esophageal manometry in clinical practice. *Am J Gastroenterol* 1998;93:2359-2362.

Barloon TJ, Bergus GR, Lu CC. Diagnostic imaging in the evaluation of dysphagia. *Am Fam Physician* 1996;53(2):535-546.

Bonavina L, DeMeester TR, McChesney L, et al. Drug-induced esophageal strictures. *Ann Surg* 1987;206(2):173-183.

Bremner CG. Zenker's diverticulum. *Arch Surg* 1998;133:1131-1133.

Bremner RM, DeMeester TR. Current management of patients with esophageal motor abnormalities. *Adv Surg* 1996;30:349-384.

Cook IJ, Kahrilas PJ. American Gastroenterological Association technical review on management of oropharyngeal dysphagia. *Gastroenterology* 1999;116:455-478.

DeVault KR. Lower esophageal (Schatzki's) ring: pathogenesis, diagnosis and therapy. *Dig Dis* 1996;14:323-329.

Lagergren J, Bergström R, Lindgren A, et al. Symptomatic gastroesophageal reflux as a risk factor for esophageal adenocarcinoma. *N Engl J Med* 1999;340:825-831.

Marks RD, Richter JE, Rizzo J, et al. Omeprazole versus H_2-receptor antagonists in treating patients with peptic stricture and esophagitis. *Gastroenterology* 1994;106:907-915.

Patti MG, Feo CV, DePinto M, et al. Results of laparoscopic antireflux surgery for dysphagia and gastroesophageal reflux disease. *Am J Surg* 1998;176:564-568.

Spiess AE, Kahrilas PJ. Treating achalasia: from whalebone to laparoscope. *JAMA* 1998;280:638-642.

CHAPTER 9

Heartburn

Mitchell King

DEFINITION

Heartburn is a retrosternal burning sensation radiating upward toward the neck, generally caused by a reflux of gastric acid into the esophagus. However, patients may use the term "heartburn" to describe a variety of symptoms associated with several different disease processes. Therefore, a detailed history and a focused physical examination are critical in directing the evaluation and treatment of this common symptom.

CLINICAL MANIFESTATIONS

Heartburn is a common patient complaint, experienced by up to 40% of patients at least once per month and by 7% on a daily basis. The clinical presentation and associated symptoms encompass a wide spectrum of disorders—from heartburn without esophagitis to severe complications such as stricture, bleeding, and metaplasia of the esophageal mucosa. Although typically not a life-threatening disorder, heartburn can be a chronic problem that has a significant effect on a patient's quality of life.

Heartburn with regurgitation is the classic presentation for gastroesophageal reflux disease (GERD). The regurgitation symptoms may be referred to as "water brash" or an acidic taste in the throat that consists of acidic material and small amounts of undigested food.

Atypical chest pain. In addition to the typical heartburn symptoms, many patients experience chest pain as a manifestation of GERD. Chest pain from GERD can be difficult to distinguish from a cardiac cause. Cardiovascular evaluation, including electrocardiography and stress testing, may be needed before testing for a gastrointestinal cause.

Respiratory symptoms. Regurgitation, particularly at night, can be a potential cause for laryngitis, recurrent pneumonia, and nonseasonal asthma. GERD should be considered in the differential diagnosis of these conditions.

Dysphagia can occur in association with gastroesophageal reflux. In addition, reflux can cause inflammatory and cellular changes (Barrett's esophagus) that can lead to the development of structural lesions such as a stricture or carcinoma, both of which can also cause dysphagia. Esophageal motility disorders, extrinsic compression from other structures, connective tissue disease, and neuromuscular diseases are other potential causes for dysphagia (see Chapter 8).

Heartburn with gastrointestinal (GI) bleeding. Gastrointestinal bleeding can occur with severe esophagitis. However, gastroesophageal bleeding presenting with anemia, unstable vital signs, hematemesis, or melena generally is more consistent with either peptic ulcer disease or a colonic lesion as the underlying cause for GI bleeding. Esophageal varices or Mallory-Weiss tears are additional causes of GI bleeding.

Heartburn with abdominal pain. Many causes are found for abdominal pain. When heartburn is a significant symptom along with the abdominal pain, peptic ulcer disease, gastroesophageal reflux, cholecystitis, and non-ulcer dyspepsia are potential causes. Significant upper abdominal pain with rigidity, rebound tenderness, and fever suggests cholecystitis, pancreatitis, or peptic ulcer (with penetration) as potential causes.

PATIENT HISTORY

Initial evaluation of the patient presenting with a complaint of heartburn includes the patient's detailed description of the episodes along with assessment of risk for the different diseases with heartburn as a presenting symptom. Table 9.1 outlines important elements of the history.

Description of symptoms. Burning pain in the epigastric, sternal, and throat regions brought on by being in the recumbent position or bending over, in association with regurgitation of gastric contents, is most characteristic of GERD. Burning, aching, or gnawing pain in the epigastric region or upper quadrants of the abdomen is typical of peptic ulcer disease. Chest tightness, rather than burning, is more typical of cardiac disease. Colicky upper abdominal pain is indicative of cholecystitis, nephrolithiasis, irritable bowel syndrome, or non-ulcer dyspepsia.

Relationship to meals. Table 9.2 lists factors that can bring on or worsen heartburn associated with gastroesophageal reflux. The pain of esophageal reflux may be alleviated by antacids or consumption of food or liquids, but frequently recurs within 1 to 2 hours. Peptic ulcer disease is often described as being associated with hunger pains, and can be relieved by eating. Commonly, the pain of peptic ulcer disease is more intense in the middle of the night and is more typically midepigastric in location. Pain brought on by exertion and relieved by rest suggests a cardiac cause. Cholecystitis is usually aggravated by eating, and the pain of nephrolithiasis is independent of food ingestion. Irritable bowel syndrome pain is brought on by eating and relieved by passage of a bowel movement. The pain of non-ulcer dyspepsia is more variable, but often related to eating.

Associated intestinal symptoms. Heartburn, regurgitation, and dysphagia are the most common symptoms of gastroesophageal reflux, although nausea may also occur. Nausea and vomiting are symptoms consistent with peptic ulcer disease, non-ulcer dyspepsia, cholecystitis, or nephrolithiasis. Alteration between loose stools and constipation suggests irritable bowel syndrome as a potential cause. Melena or hematochezia points toward peptic ulcer disease or a colonic lesion.

T ABLE 9.1. Important historical elements to evaluate in patients with heartburn

Description of symptoms
Timing in relation to meals
Associated intestinal symptoms
Associated extra-intestinal symptoms
Fever
Weight loss
Medications
Past medical and surgical history
Family history
Smoking history
Dietary history

T ABLE 9.2.   Factors that can worsen heartburn associated with reflux disease

Being in the supine position
Eating large meals
Smoking cigarettes, cigars, or pipes
Drinking caffeinated beverages or alcohol
Eating citrus fruits, tomato-based products, chocolate, mints, fatty foods, onions, or spicy foods
Taking certain medications (see Table 9.3)

Associated extraintestinal symptoms. GERD can also cause respiratory symptoms of cough, wheezing, sore throat, and laryngitis. Heartburn associated with shortness of breath and chest pain should raise concerns about a cardiac cause of the patient's symptoms.

Fever. Presence of fever suggests the possibility of the patient's symptoms being caused by cholecystitis, pancreatitis, nephrolithiasis with secondary infection, or penetration of a peptic ulcer. Pneumonia should also be considered, although heartburn would be an uncommon presenting complaint. Patients with human immunodeficiency virus (HIV) infection or patients undergoing chemotherapy can have fevers caused by infectious esophagitis. *Candida*, cytomegalovirus, and herpes simplex are the most common pathogens.

Weight loss. Although weight loss can occur with nonmalignant causes of heartburn symptoms, significant weight loss raises concern about an underlying malignancy. Patients with HIV can have weight loss associated with esophagitis, and they will commonly have significant weight loss as HIV progresses.

Medications. Certain medications can precipitate or exacerbate symptoms associated with GERD (Table 9.3). Nonsteroidal antiinflammatory drugs (NSAIDs) are associated with gastric and duodenal ulcers, as well as heartburn. Any medications

T ABLE 9.3.   Medications that may exacerbate gastroesophageal reflux disease

NSAIDs
Tetracycline
Alendronate (Fosamax)
Quinidine
Potassium chloride
Iron
Progesterone
Theophylline
Anticholinergic agents
β–adrenergic agonists
α–adrenergic antagonists
Benzodiazepines
Nitrates
Calcium channel blockers

NSAIDs, nonsteroidal antiinflammatory drugs.

the patient is using to alleviate symptoms should also be elicited, particularly with the availability of over-the-counter (OTC) histamine$_2$ (H$_2$) blockers.

Medical and surgical history. History of previously diagnosed gastrointestinal diseases can aid in directing the evaluation. Monitoring illnesses linked with heartburn symptoms (e.g., asthma) may be helpful in treating the patient. Connective tissue and neuromuscular disease can be underlying causes for esophageal symptoms.

Family history is not a known risk factor for gastroesophageal reflux, but may be for peptic ulcer disease, either by virtue of common exposure to *Helicobacter pylori* or similar habits regarding the use of NSAIDs and tobacco.

Smoking history. In addition to its association with cardiac disease, smoking can worsen gastroesophageal reflux and is a risk factor for peptic ulcer disease.

Dietary history. Dietary factors associated with gastroesophageal reflux are listed in Table 9.2. No specific dietary correlates are seen for peptic ulcer disease. However, alcohol can cause gastric irritation with resultant gastritis.

PHYSICAL EXAMINATION

The physical examination generally cannot distinguish between gastritis, peptic ulcer disease, non-ulcer dyspepsia, and GERD. All of these typically have minimal physical findings other than epigastric tenderness. A hemoccult test may show evidence of blood loss. If blood loss occurs, then peptic ulcer disease and erosive gastritis or esophagitis are the more likely diagnoses than simple gastroesophageal reflux.

Cardiac findings such as S_3, S_4, pulmonary rales, or irregular rhythm signify underlying cardiac disease. Abdominal tenderness with pancreatitis is typically periumbilical, whereas the tenderness with cholecystitis is in the right upper quadrant, is associated with a positive Murphy's sign, and may be accompanied by jaundice. Nephrolithiasis typically presents no physical findings other than possible costovertebral angle tenderness. Palpation of a mass suggests the presence of a neoplasm.

DIAGNOSTIC STUDIES

No single test is accepted as the standard for diagnosing GERD. However, several tests may prove useful in evaluating patients with heartburn.

Esophagogastroduodenoscopy (EGD) is the diagnostic tool most frequently used in evaluating the symptoms of heartburn or dysphagia and in assessing the upper gastrointestinal tract in patients with GI blood loss. EGD will detect esophagitis, erosions, ulcerations, malignancies, webs, diverticula, and strictures, and it can be therapeutically useful in treating ulcer disease and strictures.

Barium studies can be useful in detecting anatomic abnormalities and esophageal spasm, and they may detect reflux. However, barium studies have a lower sensitivity than EGD for detecting ulcerations, erosions, and tumors, and they do not allow tissue diagnosis.

Ambulatory esophageal pH monitoring. For this test, a thin pH probe is placed through the patient's nose into the esophagus 5 cm above the lower esophageal sphincter. The percentage of time the esophageal pH is below 4, in conjunction with the patient's symptoms, is used as diagnostic information. The reported sensitivity and specificity for this test are both 95%. However, for most patients with typical symptoms, this test is not necessary. Its primary role would be to evaluate patients with atypical symptoms, normal endoscopy, or those refractory to therapy.

The **acid perfusion test** involves perfusion of hydrochloric acid via a nasogastric tube into the esophagus. It has a high specificity but low sensitivity and is no longer commonly used because of the availability of endoscopy and pH monitoring.

Esophageal manometry involves monitoring of lower esophageal sphincter pressures and esophageal peristalsis. Its primary role is to evaluate patients for motility disorders.

Helicobacter pylori testing is outlined in Table 9.4.

Rapid urease test. This test analyzes tissue samples obtained during endoscopy for the presence of urease. The presence of urease is consistent with *H. pylori* infection. This test has a sensitivity of approximately 90% and a specificity of 98%. The test itself is inexpensive and quickly performed, but obtaining samples is expensive because of the costs associated with endoscopy. This is the most commonly relied on test for diagnosing *H. pylori* in patients with gastritis or ulcers who undergo endoscopy.

Histologic staining. If the rapid urease test is negative in a patient with ulcers or gastritis, then a separate sample can be sent for histologic staining for the presence of *H. pylori*. Histologic staining has excellent sensitivity and specificity; however, it is slower and more expensive than the urease test.

Serologic tests have the advantage of being noninvasive, inexpensive, and highly sensitive and specific (> 90%). The disadvantages are that serology will remain indefinitely positive, and a positive test indicates only prior infection—not necessarily current activity. Patients in their 20s are rarely positive, whereas those in their 60s are positive more than 50% of the time. This test can be useful in younger patients and for diagnosing *H. pylori* in radiographically diagnosed duodenal ulcers; it cannot, however, be relied on in older patients with gastric ulcers or to follow therapeutic response.

Breath tests involve having the patient ingest urea labeled with radioactive carbon. If *H. pylori* is present, urease hydrolyzes the urea and the patient exhales labeled carbon dioxide. The test is both sensitive and specific, but is not readily available. In the future, this test will likely become the test of choice to document eradication of *H. pylori* infection because it is noninvasive and less expensive than tests requiring endoscopy.

T ABLE 9.4. Diagnostic tests for *helicobacter pylori*

Test	Costs	Comments
Rapid urease test	$$$	The test itself is inexpensive but requires endoscopy
		Results promptly obtained
		Sensitive/very specific
Histologic staining/culture	$$$	Requires endoscopy
		Takes longer to receive results
		More expensive than rapid urease test
Serology	$	Noninvasive
		Inexpensive
		Documents exposure but not active disease
		Cannot document eradication
Urea breath tests	$/$$	Noninvasive
		Variable cost but can be inexpensive
		Sensitive/specific
		Can document eradication

$, least expensive; $$, intermediate cost; $$$, most expensive.

RISK FACTORS

Drinking alcohol and caffeinated beverages and smoking decrease lower esophageal sphincter pressure, predisposing the patient to gastroesophageal reflux. Smoking may also play a role in development of *H. pylori*-negative peptic ulcer disease. Alcohol causes gastric irritation and erosive gastritis.

Obesity and pregnancy may promote reflux by increasing the intraabdominal pressure at the gastroesophageal junction.

Medications (Table 9.3) can contribute to GERD. In addition, NSAIDs are the leading cause of *H. pylori*-negative peptic ulcer disease.

Immunocompromised states, such as cancer, organ transplant, and HIV infection, put patients at higher risk for developing infectious esophagitis.

Stress, both physical and emotional, is associated with peptic ulcer disease.

Dietary factors associated with the development of GERD are listed in Table 9.2.

PATHOPHYSIOLOGY

The most common gastrointestinal causes for heartburn symptoms are GERD, peptic ulcer disease, gastritis, and non-ulcer dyspepsia. Symptoms overlap with each of these entities, but each has a different pathophysiologic basis.

Gastroesophageal reflux occurs when reflux or regurgitation of gastric contents (which are acidic in nature) enter the esophagus. Decreased lower esophageal sphincter pressure or increased intraabdominal pressure play a significant role in this process. The low pH of the gastric contents causes inflammatory changes leading to esophagitis. Continued acid exposure can cause the normal squamous cells lining the distal esophagus to undergo adenomatous metaplastic transformation (Barrett's esophagus). This adenomatous tissue can then undergo transformation to become esophageal adenocarcinoma. Patients with Barrett's esophagus are at a higher risk (30 to 40 times) for developing esophageal cancer. Continued inflammatory reaction can also lead to scarring within the esophagus and to the development of a stricture with resultant dysphagia. *H. pylori* has not yet been identified to have a role in GERD.

Peptic ulcer disease and the more common forms of gastritis have similar symptoms, causes, and risk factors. Peptic ulcer disease occurs in 5% to 10% of people at some time in their lives. Peptic ulcer disease tends to be recurrent and to occur more commonly in older patients and in men. Risk factors for the development of peptic ulcers and gastritis have been identified. Typically, the gastric and duodenal mucosa are resistant to any damage from acid secretion. Peptic ulcers and gastritis occur when the defense mechanisms are compromised or, rarely, when acid secretion is sufficient to overwhelm the defenses.

The most significant risk factor for the development of peptic ulcer disease is *H. pylori* infection. Gastric infection with *H. pylori* causes gastritis. In 10% to 20% of infected individuals, gastric or duodenal ulcers develop. Exactly why peptic ulcers occur and why the ulcers are more prevalent in the duodenum is unclear. Infection with *H. pylori* is also associated with the development of gastric adenocarcinoma and gastric lymphoma.

NSAIDs contribute to gastritis and ulcer formation by blocking cyclooxygenase-1 production of prostaglandins that maintain mucosal blood flow, mucus secretion, and bicarbonate. Without these protective factors, acid-induced inflammation and ulcers may result. Stress-induced gastritis and ulcers are thought to occur from impaired mucosal defense resulting from vasoconstriction and resultant tissue hypoxia.

Non-ulcer dyspepsia is a poorly understood disease with symptoms like those of GERD and peptic ulcer disease, but with no identifiable abnormality on testing.

The pathophysiology is thought to be that of altered GI motility and contractile patterns.

DIFFERENTIAL DIAGNOSIS

Table 9.5 presents a comprehensive differential diagnosis for patients with heartburn complaints. The most common causes for heartburn symptoms are GERD, peptic ulcer disease, gastritis, and non-ulcer dyspepsia.

Gastroesophageal reflux symptoms of heartburn are experienced on a daily basis by 7% of the population, on a weekly basis by 15%, and at least monthly by up to 40%. The classic symptoms of gastroesophageal reflux are heartburn and regurgitation of acidic and food materials.

Patients with typical gastroesophageal reflux symptoms of heartburn and regurgitation can undergo empirical treatment with lifestyle modifications and acid suppressive therapy without diagnostic evaluation (Tables 9.6 and 9.7). If the patient fails to respond to therapy within 6 weeks, then a diagnostic evaluation is indicated. Patients with dysphagia, early satiety, emesis, bleeding, weight loss, or extraesophageal symptoms (e.g., wheezing, cough, laryngitis, or chest pain) should

T ABLE 9.5. Differential diagnosis of heartburn

Differential diagnosis	Typical symptoms
Gastroesophageal reflux disease	Regurgitation, dysphagia
Peptic ulcer disease	Gnawing epigastric pain, nausea, vomiting, bloating
Gastritis	Same as peptic ulcer disease
Nonulcer dyspepsia	Upper abdominal/epigastric pain, bloating, belching, flatulence, nausea
Coronary artery disease/angina	Chest pressure, nausea, diaphoresis, palpitations
Cholelithiasis	Colicky right upper quadrant pain, with meals; radiation to scapular region
Pancreatitis	Severe constant midabdominal pain
Infectious esophagitis	Dysphagia, associated immunocompromised condition
Medication or chemical esophagitis	Dysphagia, associated ingestion
Scleroderma/polymyositis with secondary gastroesophageal reflux	Associated signs of connective tissue disease, potential risk of stricture/dysphagia

T ABLE 9.6. Behavioral modification for treatment of gastroesophageal reflux disease

Cease food or beverage ingestion for 2 to 3 h before reclining
Lose weight, if overweight
Avoid overeating
Avoid tight restrictive clothing
Elevate head of bed with blocks (4–6 inches)
Eat a high-protein, low-fat diet
Avoid specific foods and medications that may exacerbate gastroesophageal reflux disease (Tables 9.2 and 9.3)

TABLE 9.7. Medication therapy for gastroesophageal reflux disease and peptic ulcer disease

	Cost	Usual dosage		Side effects
		GERD TX/ Maintenance	PUD TX/ Maintenance	
Antacids[a]	$	qid, 1 h after meals and bedtime		Varies with antacid, belching, nausea altered bowel habits, and flatulence; alkaluria (nephrolithiasis), hypercalcemia, hypermagnesemia, and alkalosis
H$_2$ Receptor Blockers				
Cimetidine (Tagamet)	$$	800 mg bid/ 400 mg bid	800 mg qd/ 400 mg qd	Headache, dizziness, nausea, myalgia, skin rash, itching, GI disturbance CNS changes can occur, especially in the elderly Rare reports of blood dyscrasias and hepatitis Long-term use: loss of libido, impotence, gynecomastia Inhibits hepatic enzymes causing multiple drug interactions
Famotidine (Pepcid)	$$	40 mg bid/20 mg bid	40 mg qd/20 mg qd	Headache, dizziness, GI disturbance, somnolence, depression; rarely, seizures and palpitations
Nizatidine (Axid)	$$	300 mg bid/ 150 mg bid	300 mg qd/ 150 mg qd	Anemia, dizziness, sweating, and urticaria

Drug	Cost	Dose	Dose	Side Effects/Comments
Ranitidine (Zantac)	$$	300 mg bid (or 150 mg qid)/150 mg bid	300 mg qd/150 mg qd	Headache, rash, GI disturbance, hepatitis, CNS disturbance; rarely: arthralgia, myalgia, blood dyscrasia, arrhythmia, anaphylaxis and angioneurotic edema; caution with alcohol
Proton Pump Inhibitors				
Lansoprazole (Prevacid)	$$$	15–30 mg qd/15 mg qd	15–30 mg qd/15 mg qd	Nausea, diarrhea, and abdominal pain
Omeprazole (Prilosec)	$$$	20 mg qd/20 mg qd	20–40 mg qd/20 mg qd	Headache, GI disturbance, rash, dizziness, cough, and abdominal pain
Prokinetic Agents				
Cisapride (Propulsid)[b]	$$$	10 mg qid	N/A	Headache, GI disturbance, rhinitis, pain, abnormal vision, and arrhythmias. Should not be given to patients with chest pain related to heart disease, with arrhythmias, or with other cardiovascular problems
Metoclopramide (Reglan)	$	5–10 mg qid	N/A	Restlessness, fatigue, parkinsonism, tardive dyskinesia, neuroleptic malignant syndrome, dizziness, hyper- or hypotension, and GI upset

[a]Not FDA approved for GERD or peptic ulcer disease.

[b]Because of concerns about heart rhythm abnormalities, Cisapride is expected to be voluntarily withdrawn from the U.S. market in mid-2000. At press time, Cisapride was available for limited use.

bid, twice daily; CNS, central nervous system; FDA, Food and Drug Administration; GERD, gastroesophageal reflux disease; GI, gastrointestinal; N/A, not applicable; PUD, peptic ulcer dispose; qd, every day; qid, four times daily; TX, treatment.

$, least expensive; $$, intermediate cost; $$$, most expensive.

undergo diagnostic evaluation without delay. Gastrointestinal evaluation usually involves endoscopy, but it also can include barium studies for patients with dysphagia. Up to 30% of patients with gastroesophageal reflux will have normal esophageal mucosa at endoscopy. In patients with normal endoscopic findings who are also refractory to therapy, further diagnostic testing with pH monitoring or motility studies may be indicated.

Peptic ulcer disease is present in 1.5% of the population and will occur in up to 10% of the population at some time during their lifetime. Duodenal ulcers occur more commonly than gastric ulcers, and they also begin to occur at a younger age. Men are affected by peptic ulcer disease slightly more than women. More than half of ulcer patients have symptoms for more than 2 years before they seek treatment. Without treatment, 30% or more of patients will experience healing of their disease over a 4 to 12 week period, but 75% to 80% will have a recurrence.

Symptoms consistent with peptic ulcer disease are a mild-to-moderate upper abdominal (usually epigastric) gnawing or burning pain relieved by eating or taking antacids. The pain can be described as heartburn, and can be associated with other abdominal complaints such as nausea, vomiting, bloating, or belching. Significant acute abdominal pain suggests complications of penetration or perforation. In patients aged less than 40 years with symptoms consistent with uncomplicated peptic ulcer disease and who are negative for occult bleeding, an *H. pylori* serologic test can be used to direct therapy. In older patients and patients aged less than 40 years with refractory symptoms, endoscopy is generally required to make the diagnosis. Pathology and testing of any tissue samples for *H. pylori* will direct therapy.

Acute gastritis, gastric ulcers, and duodenal ulcers present with indistinguishable symptoms. Heartburn is one of the symptoms with which the patient may present. Causes of gastritis are listed in Table 9.8. The diagnosis of gastritis can be made with the same process as described above for peptic ulcer disease.

Non-ulcer dyspepsia is a poorly understood disease with symptoms overlapping GERD, peptic ulcer disease, and gastritis. Non-ulcer dyspepsia occurs in up to 25% to 30% of the population at some time in their lives. This is generally considered a diagnosis of exclusion. In patients aged less than 45 years in whom the initial laboratory evaluation (complete blood count, hemoccult testing of the stools, *H. pylori* serology) is normal, empiric therapy can be undertaken based on the patient's predominant symptoms. For patients whose symptoms are predominantly heartburn and reflux, choose acid suppressive therapy, whereas for patients whose symptoms are consis-

---

T ABLE 9.8.   Causes of gastritis

Stress

Medications

Mechanical trauma (e.g., nasogastric tubes)

Ischemia

Helicobacter pylori infection

Autoimmune

Other infections: tuberculosis, syphilis, cytomegalovirus, herpes, candida, histoplasma, cryptococcus, aspergillus, cryptosporidiosis, other parasites

Crohn's disease

Sarcoidosis

Idiopathic

tent with delayed emptying, choose prokinetic agents. Patients presenting after age 45 require more aggressive evaluation because organic disease becomes more prevalent as the patients get older.

REFERRAL

Referral to a specialist is generally indicated for those patients who require endoscopy and for those with refractory symptoms in whom the diagnosis is uncertain. For example, esophageal infection with opportunistic infections such as cytomegalovirus, herpes, or *Candida* can cause heartburn. Endoscopy, with tissue samples for culture and microscopy, particularly in immunocompromised patients, confirms the diagnosis. Treat patients with typical gastroesophageal reflux symptoms empirically. Younger patients with symptoms consistent with peptic ulcer disease or gastritis can be tested for *H. pylori* antibodies and treated based on this testing. These patients and patients with non-ulcer dyspepsia should be referred only if therapy is unsuccessful. More aggressive approaches are warranted in patients aged more than 45 years, and earlier referrals are often indicated. Table 9.9 presents signs and symptoms that may signify the need for earlier referral.

Surgical referral may be indicated for patients with GERD who are nonresponsive to maximal medical therapy, or who have recurrent ulceration, bleeding, strictures, or Barrett's esophagus.

Hospitalization may be required for patients presenting with GI bleeding and anemia, depending on the patient's age, other medical problems, and current vital signs. In patients with nausea or vomiting, dehydration or electrolyte abnormalities may dictate the need for hospitalization. Patients presenting with chest pain may require admission to eliminate cardiac disease as the underlying cause. Patients with asthma-type symptoms or pneumonia may require hospitalization to treat their lung disease.

MANAGEMENT

The spectrum of GERD ranges from minimal symptoms and objective findings to severe disease with associated complications such as stricture, bleeding, or Barrett's esophagus. Therapy should be tailored to the patient. Initial therapy for mild GERD may involve behavioral or lifestyle modifications (Tables 9.6 and 9.7, Figure 9.1), along with over-the-counter H_2 blockers or antacids. In patients who have already tried these agents or are unresponsive to them, use prescription-strength H_2 blockers, proton pump inhibitors, or motility agents, along with continued reinforcement of lifestyle modifications. If symptoms are relieved, then initiate maintenance therapy. Symptoms persisting beyond 6 weeks merit referral for endoscopy.

T ABLE 9.9. Indications for gastroenterology referral in heartburn patients

Dysphagia
Evidence of bleeding
Early satiety
Recurrent vomiting
Weight loss
Atypical symptoms
Diagnostic uncertainty
Refractory to therapy

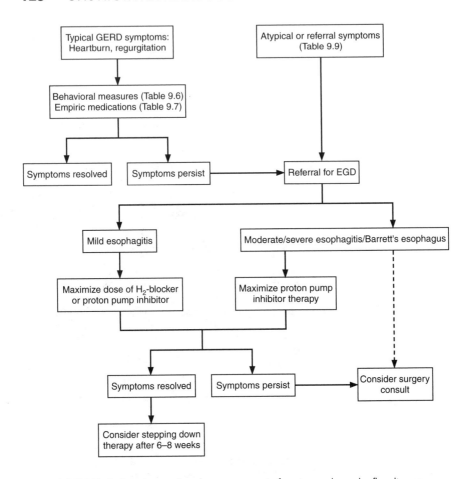

FIGURE 9.1. Approach to the management of gastroesophageal reflux disease.

The rate of recurrence with GERD is very high because the underlying patho-physiologic process is unchanged when therapy is discontinued. Therapy for moderate to severe esophagitis and atypical symptoms, particularly respiratory, may require long-term treatment. Nonetheless, attempt to step down therapy after 8 weeks of symptom control. Some patients may require only intermittent therapy along with continued lifestyle modifications. Severe esophagitis, Barrett's esophagus, and stricture are markers of severe reflux and require long-term treatment, even in the absence of symptoms, to reduce the risk of esophageal carcinoma, bleeding, or disease progression.

Therapy for **peptic ulcer disease and gastritis** is dependent on the patient's status regarding the presence of *H. pylori* infection. If *H. pylori* is present, then therapy directed against this organism is indicated (Table 9.10). After completion of the antibiotic regimen, proton pump inhibitors are generally continued for 4 to 8 weeks for duodenal ulcers and for 6 to 12 weeks for gastritis or gastric ulcers.

T ABLE 9.10. Therapy for peptic ulcer disease

Therapy	Comments
Helicobacter pylori-Positive Ulcer	
Omeprazole (Prilosec), 40 mg qd	7-day regimen, 90% to 95% effective
Clarithromycin (Biaxin), 500 mg tid	Continue proton pump inhibitors for 4–8 weeks for
Ampicillin[a] (Principen), 500 mg or	duodenal ulcers, and 6–12 weeks for gastritis or
OR	gastric ulcers
Metronidazole (Flagyl), 250 mg qid	Follow-up endoscopy to document healing of gastric
	ulcers
Ranitidine (Zantac), 150 mg bid	14-day regimen, 80% to 85% effective
Bismuth subsalicylate (Pepto-Bismol), 2 tablets qid	Two-thirds the cost of above regimen
Metronidazole (Flagyl), 250 mg qid	Duration of acid suppression with ranitidine and
Tetracycline, 500 mg qid	follow-up endoscopy as above
H. pylori-Negative Ulcers	
H$_2$ receptor Blockers	Misoprostal (Cytotec), 200 μg qid useful for
Cimetidine (Tagamet), 800 mg qhs or	preventing NSAID-related ulcers
400 mg bid	Sucralfate (Carafate) antacids or intravenous H$_2$
Ranitidine (Zantac), 300 mg qhs or 150 mg bid	blockers may help prevent stress ulcers in critically
Nizatidine (Axid), 300 mg qhs or 150 mg bid	ill patients
Famotidine (Pepcid), 40 mg qhs or 20 mg bid	Duration of therapy and indications for follow-up
Proton Pump Inhibitors	endoscopy as above for *H. pylori*-positive patients
Omeprazole (Prilosec), 20 mg qd	Higher doses required for hypersecretory states (e.g.,
Lansoprazole (Prevacid), 15 mg qd	Zollinger-Ellison)

[a]Not approved by the US Food and Drug Administration for this use.

bid, twice daily; NSAID, nonsteroidal antiinflammatory drug; qd, every day; qid, four times daily; tid, three times daily.

Patients with **NSAID-related ulcers** are generally treated with acid suppression therapy and discontinuance of the NSAID. If NSAIDs must be used, options include switching the patient to a nonacetylated salicylate, such as salsalate (Disalcid), using an enterically coated preparation, and prescribing the lowest effective dose. Ulcer healing should be documented before stopping acid suppression therapy. If NSAIDs must be used in patients with a history of ulcer, misoprostal (Cytotec) can help prevent recurrence. Another option is to use a COX-2 inhibitor such as rofecoxib (Vioxx) or celecoxib (Celebrex).

Therapy for **non-ulcer dyspepsia** involves avoidance of precipitating foods or medications, reassurance regarding the absence of serious disease, and medications directed at the predominant symptoms. In patients with ulcerlike or reflux symptoms, acid-suppressing agents can be used. In patients with dysmotility-related symptoms (e.g., nausea, bloating, or early satiety), try motility agents (Table 9.7). If treatment is initially successful, try 4 weeks of continuous therapy and then a trial without medication. Some patients benefit from intermittent therapy, whereas others require continuous treatment. In such cases, periodic trials without medication should be attempted to see if medication is still necessary.

FOLLOW-UP

Follow-up for most patients with **gastroesophageal reflux** involves assessing symptom relief. After 6 to 8 weeks, consider stepping down therapy, with subsequent trials without medications. Some patients may require long-term or intermittent therapy for symptom control. Patients with refractory symptoms will need further diagnostic evaluation. Patients found to have severe esophagitis or Barrett's esophagus at endoscopy are at increased risk for esophageal cancer. These patients will require long-term therapy and follow-up endoscopy every 6 to 24 months, depending on the presence and grade of dysplasia.

Patients with **stricture formation** should be questioned regarding the presence of dysphagia. If present, then endoscopic dilatation may provide symptomatic relief. Long-term proton pump inhibitor therapy has been shown to help prevent stricture progression.

Patients with **gastric ulcers** require follow-up endoscopy before stopping therapy because gastric carcinomas can have the appearance of a gastric ulcer, and biopsy specimens may not identify the carcinoma. Patients with duodenal ulcers can be assessed for resolution of symptoms or correction of anemia. Patients with peptic ulcer disease should be instructed to report any recurrence of symptoms. With recurrence, endoscopy is often indicated. In patients with previously documented *H. pylori* and symptom recurrence within 2 years of therapy, urea breath testing can be performed to assess for the presence of *H. pylori*. If present, prescribe therapy to eradicate *H. pylori*.

Follow-up for patients with **non-ulcer dyspepsia** involves inquiry into symptom relief and reassurance regarding the diagnosis and nonserious nature of this condition. After completion of the initial workup, further testing is usually not indicated unless new symptoms develop.

PATIENT EDUCATION

Patient education about **GERD** should focus on an explanation of what is causing the symptoms, how various factors can influence the occurrence of symptoms, and things the patient can do to minimize symptom occurrence (Table 9.6). In addition, also advise the patient to report new symptoms, particularly bleeding, melena, emesis, dysphagia, or respiratory complaints.

Patient education for **peptic ulcer disease and gastritis** can be divided into two approaches: For those who are *H. pylori* positive, emphasize the importance of compliance with and completion of drug therapy. For patients who are *H. pylori* negative, stress the role various substances (e.g., NSAIDs and smoking) have in their disease along with strong advice to avoid precipitating factors. For follow-up, also inquire into symptom relief and development of new symptoms and stress the importance of following through with any recommended repeat endoscopic procedures.

Patients with **non-ulcer dyspepsia** need reassurance about the "realness" of this disease that has no concrete findings. Describe the pathophysiology, prevalence, and lack of serious long-term consequences, which should be helpful to patients. In addition, help the patient identify precipitating factors, advise avoidance of these factors, and offer medical therapy directed at the predominant symptoms.

SUGGESTED READING

Ament PW, Childers RS. Prophylaxis and treatment of NSAID-induced gastropathy. *Am Fam Physician* 1997;55:1323–1326, 1331–1332.

Fass R, Hixson LJ, Ciccolo ML, et al. Contemporary medical therapy for gastroesophageal reflux disease. *Am Fam Physician* 1997;55: 205-212, 217-218.

Feldman M. Peptic ulcer diseases. In: Dale DC, Federman DD, eds. *Scientific American medicine*. New York: Scientific American, 1999.

Kahrilas PJ. Gastroesophageal reflux disease. *JAMA* 1996;276:983-988.

Pezzi JS, Shiau YF. *Helicobacter pylori* and gastrointestinal disease. *Am Fam Physician* 1995;52:1717-1724, 1729.

Talley NJ. Nonulcer dyspepsia: current approaches to diagnosis and management. *Am Fam Physician* 1993;47:1407-1416.

Young HS. Esophageal disorders. In: Dale DC, Federman DD, eds. *Scientific American medicine*. New York: Scientific American, 1999.

CHAPTER 10

··

Abdominal Masses in Children

Mari E. Egan

DEFINITION

Abdominal masses found in children are usually asymptomatic and are typically first discovered by the parents during bathing or by physicians as part of a routine physical examination. Palpable abdominal masses are the most frequent finding of malignant solid tumors in children. Although a variety of benign entities present as abdominal masses, any mass requires evaluation to rule out a malignancy. The following discussion emphasizes the more common abdominal tumors seen in infants and children: neuroblastoma, Wilms' tumor, and hepatic neoplasms.

CLINICAL MANIFESTATIONS

When obtaining a history and performing a physical examination it is important to detect whether a discrete abdominal mass exists and whether symptoms are referable to the mass. Abdominal enlargement can be caused by a neoplasm, as well as by diminished wall musculature tone, increased fluid content (ascites, full bladder), increased gas (intestinal obstruction, perforated viscus), stool (constipation), a solid mass (hepatomegaly, renal cysts), or pregnancy.

Age

The age of a patient is a helpful clue. Table 10.1 lists the most common abdominal tumors by age. Age is an especially important consideration in young children because a wide variation is seen in rates of specific childhood cancers by age. Neuroblastoma is by far the most commonly diagnosed neoplasm in the first year of life. The average age for occurrence of Wilms' tumor is 3 to 4 years of age, and it is the most common abdominal malignancy. In older children, a mass is more likely to be secondary to leukemia or lymphoma with involvement of the liver and spleen. Rhabdomyosarcoma has a bimodal curve with a initial peak at age 3 to 5 years and a later peak around age 15 to 19 years. It is not uncommon for a rhabdomyosarcoma of the genitourinary tract to present as an abdominal mass. Age is also important in predicting the survival rate after treatment. In neuroblastoma, age is an important independent variable to determine outcome. Children aged younger than 1 year have significantly better survival rates than older children.

Presenting Symptoms

Most children with abdominal tumors are asymptomatic, and the tumors are usually discovered when parents or physicians detect a mass or increased abdominal girth. In taking the history, it is important to inquire about symptoms related to the abdominal mass. Because many abdominal masses are related to the renal system, it is important to elicit a thorough genitourinary history.

T ABLE 10.1. Common malignant pediatric abdominal tumors by age

NEWBORN (<1 Y)
Neuroblastoma
Wilms' tumor (>6 months)
Hepatoblastoma
Mesoblastic nephroma

INFANTS (1–3 Y)
Neuroblastoma
Wilms' tumor
Hepatoblastoma
Leukemia

CHILD (3–11 Y)
Wilms' tumor
Lymphoma
Neuroblastoma
Hepatoblastoma
Rhabdomyosarcoma

ADOLESCENT/YOUNG ADULT (12–21 Y)
Lymphoma
Hepatocellular carcinoma
Rhabdomyosarcoma

Signs and Symptoms

Signs and symptoms vary with the site of the primary tumor, presence or absence of local spread or distant metastases, and the presence of endocrine activity. Table 10.2 lists some of the other signs and symptoms that may be seen with the three most common abdominal tumors.

PHYSICAL EXAMINATION

In a child with a suspicious abdominal mass, a thorough abdominal examination is essential but not always easy. Diverting the child's attention with an older sibling or using a pacifier or bottle may allow the child to relax and make an adequate examination possible. It is important to remember that the liver, spleen, kidneys, aorta, colon, and spine may be palpable in normal children. When the physician suspects that fecal retention is the cause of the abdominal mass, a reexamination of the child after an enema may be diagnostic. Similarly, a distended bladder causing a palpable mass may be resolved by catheterization. A rectal examination must be performed. Vaginal and pelvic examinations may be necessary in girls and adolescent women.

Neuroblastoma

Neuroblastoma arises from the malignant growth of precursors of the sympathetic nervous system. These primitive pluripotential sympathetic cells are derived from the neural crest and provide tissue found in the brain, mediastinum, adrenal medulla, pelvis, and sympathetic ganglia. Therefore, neuroblastoma can occur at any of these

T ABLE 10.2.   Other signs and symptoms of common abdominal tumors

NEUROBLASTOMA

Signs and symptoms related to tumor growth
  Pepper's syndrome—massive involvement of the liver with metastatic disease
  Superior venal cava syndrome
  Subcutaneous nodules
  Leukemoid reaction
  Hutchinson's disease—limping, bone pain, and irritability associated with bone and bone marrow metastases
  Paraplegia—extension of tumor from retroperitoneum into spinal canal
  Anemia/thrombocytopenia

SIGNS AND SYMPTOMS NOT RELATED DIRECTLY TO TUMOR GROWTH

  Horner's Syndrome—eye symptoms associated with a primary thoracic tumor
  Kerner-Morrison syndrome—intractable secretory diarrhea, vomiting, associated with a tumor that secretes
    vasoactive intestinal peptide
  Polymyoclonus-opsodonus—myoclonic jerking and random eye movements with or without cerebellar ataxia
  Failure to thrive

WILMS' TUMOR

Abdominal pain and bleeding secondary to free rupture and hemorrhage into the peritoneal cavity
Inferior vena cava thrombosis
Microscopic hematuria
Polycythemia
Anemia
Hypoglycemia
Hypertension
Weight loss
Manifestations of intravascular extension include hepatosplenomegaly, ascites, caput medusae, cardiac murmur,
    or evidence of gonadal metastasis
Varicocele—could indicate renal vein occlusion

HEPATOBLASTOMA

Mass effect symptoms—anorexia, weight loss, nausea/vomiting, abdominal pain
Elevated liver function tests
Anemia
Jaundice
Hemihypertrophy
Precocious puberty—secondary to secretion of beta human chorionic gonadotropin
Osteopenia

sites. Neuroblastoma presents as an intraabdominal tumor 50% to 70% of the time. Two-thirds of these masses are adrenal, with the remainder found in the sympathetic paraspinous ganglia. If palpable, the primary tumor is usually hard, firm, and fixed with an irregular border. The examination should assess for metastatic spread by examination for subcutaneous nodules and hepatomegaly as well as assessing signs associated with hormonal activity that can be present in neuroblastoma.

Wilms' Tumor

Wilms' tumor, a tumor of renal origin, has historically been termed "embryoma." The abdominal examination in patients with Wilms' tumor usually reveals a large, firm mass that is nontender and slightly mobile. Tenderness suggests a ruptured tumor with subcapsular or parenchymal bleeding. A rare presentation is a left-sided varicocele secondary to renal vein occlusion.

Liver Tumors

Hepatoblastoma is a solid tumor that usually arises from the right lobe of the liver. It is the most frequently occurring malignant liver tumor in children. Histologically, it is an epithelial tumor, with the epithelial cell types comprising fetal and embryonal subsets. In hepatoblastoma, the abdominal mass can be palpated as being related to the liver. The tumor is grossly large at presentation, with a pseudocapsule and areas of necrosis. Infrequently, hemihypertrophy (muscular hypertrophy of one side of the face or body) or jaundice is seen. Signs of precocious puberty secondary to secretion of β-human chorionic gonodotropin may be noted. Hepatocellular carcinoma is pathologically similar to the disease seen in adults and is an epithelial neoplasm that occurs mainly in adolescents. Rarely, it presents with signs of cirrhosis. Although size, mobility, and consistency should be noted when examining an abdominal mass, the information is not always helpful diagnostically.

DIAGNOSTIC STUDIES

Diagnostic studies should be performed to confirm the location of the mass and to characterize it (e.g., solid cystic). In the case of a potential abdominal neoplasm, the next steps are to evaluate the local tumor and vascular involvement and then to determine if metastatic disease is present. Plain films of the abdomen have been superseded by more technologically advanced procedures for evaluation of abdominal mass. Nevertheless, important information can sometimes be obtained from plain radiography. For example, neuroblastoma may reveal tumor calcifications, whereas Wilms' tumor rarely contains calcifications. Evaluation usually begins with an ultrasonographic examination of the abdomen. It is quick, inexpensive, and safe and usually does not require sedation or anesthesia. The ultrasound can usually distinguish the organ wherein the abdominal mass originated and rule out all noninvolved organ systems. In children, the retroperitoneum, liver, spleen, aorta, and inferior vena cava are typically well visualized. Ultrasound quickly differentiates solid from fluid-filled masses and directs further testing.

In suspected **neuroblastoma**, magnetic resonance imaging (MRI) is the next step because it shows full detail of the primary tumor, extension into the spinal cord, and relationship of the tumor to blood vessels and other organs. Frequently, a chest computed tomography (CT) is then performed to evaluate for lung metastasis. A new test—an "I-*meta*-iodobenzylquanidine scintigraphy (MIBG)"—is useful for evaluating possible bone or bone marrow involvement. The specific radiotype marker structurally resembles norepinephrine and is taken up in neurosecretory granules in neural crest tumors. MIBG imaging reflects the distribution of neuroblastoma in affected children. It has also been used to document recurrent disease.

Laboratory testing includes a 24-hour urine collection for catecholamine metabolites. Dopamine and norepinephrine are metabolized and secreted as vanillylmandelic acid, homovanillic acid, and metanephrine. These measurements reflect the absolute levels of tumor metabolic activity. Measurements of these metabolites are used for screening, diagnosis, and monitoring the effects of therapy. Serum studies include ferritin, neuron-specific enolase, and lactate dehydrogenase. Other biologic markers that provide staging and prognostic information are N-*myc* amplification, l-p deletion of the short arm of chromosome 1, and tumor ploidy. All of this information will be entered into a staging system to predict survival and recommend treatment.

In **Wilms' tumor**, the ultrasound will confirm the presence of a mass within the kidney as well as whether the tumor extends into the inferior vena cava or renal vein. The next test may be either a CT or MRI scan of the chest, abdomen, and pelvis. This testing further delineates renal involvement, vascular invasion, contralateral renal involvement, and lung metastases. A urinalysis is helpful because an intraoperative cystoscopy may have to be performed to exclude tumor extension into the ureter or bladder if hematuria is present.

Hepatic tumors usually appear as an echogenic mass within the liver on ultrasound examination. An abdominal MRI scan assesses the relationship of the tumor to the hepatic vasculature, and a CT scan is useful to detect pulmonary metastasis. Liver enzymes are usually normal in hepatoblastoma; however, α-fetal protein level, which is elevated in 67% of patients with hepatoblastoma, is a useful marker for evaluation of recurrences. A patient with signs of precocious puberty may have an elevated serum β–human chorionic gonadotropin level. A percutaneous needle biopsy can be used to establish the diagnosis.

Diagnostic procedures for **rhabdomyosarcoma** are ultrasound and CT scan with oral and intravenous contrast media.

Ultrasound and/or MRI and biopsy are usually needed to diagnosis **lymphoma**.

Demonstrating increased plasma or urinary levels of catecholamine yields the diagnosis of **pheochromocytoma**. Procedures to localize the tumor are CT scan, MRI, or MIBG scan.

Ultrasound is also useful for detecting conditions such as **mesoblastic nephroma, teratoma, cholededochal cysts, hydrops of the gallbladder, renal cysts, ovarian tumors, pregnancy, renal vein thrombosis**, and, in infants, **pyloric stenosis**. The ultrasound findings will guide further workup.

For suspected **nephromas, teratomas, and malignant ovarian tumors**, a biopsy is needed to confirm the diagnosis. Many clinicians will preform an upper gastrointestinal series to confirm the diagnosis of **pyloric stenosis**. Although ultrasound can usually identify benign **renal cysts**, a CT scan, intravenous pyelogram, and even a kidney biopsy may be needed to establish diagnosis with certainty.

Liver imaging using radionuclide scintigraphy and liver function tests are often useful for providing additional information in patients with **choledochal cysts**. Hormone levels are important for evaluating **ovarian masses, precocious puberty**, and **virilization**. A pregnancy test will confirm a suspected pregnancy.

For **volvulus**, plain films of the abdomen will show an abnormal intestinal gas pattern suggesting obstruction. The initial diagnosis will be confirmed by barium enema, which shows the cecum in the right upper quadrant. A barium enema is also useful for confirming the diagnosis of **intussusception**.

The diagnosis of **intestinal duplication** can be difficult. Plain films, barium studies, and ultrasound may confirm the diagnosis. Diagnosis may not be made until the time of surgery.

Ultrasound and CT scan will confirm and localize the diagnosis of **appendiceal abscess**. The white blood cell count is usually elevated with a left shift.

RISK FACTORS

Age is an important factor in the incidence of abdominal tumors as well as in prognosis. As discussed, different tumors occur with different frequency at different ages (Table 10.1).

Race is also a risk factor for some abdominal tumors. In children aged less than 1 year with neuroblastoma, the rate for whites is 64% higher than for African-Americans. Children in the racial category "other" had rates similar to African-Americans. In Wilms' tumor, African-Americans have a higher incidence rate than whites. In rhabdomyosarcoma, the incidence rate is more than four times higher in African-Americans.

Sex can be a risk factor for abdominal tumors. In neuroblastoma, little difference is seen in the incidence rate by sex. Hepatic malignancies are slightly more common in boys than in girls. In Wilms' tumor, the incidence rate for girls is higher than for boys.

Certain conditions are associated with different abdominal tumors. An association appears to exist with Beckwith-Wiedemann syndrome, hemihypertrophy, and hepatoblastoma. In families with familial adenomatous polyposis there is an increased incidence of hepatoblastoma. Wilms' tumor has been reported in association with aniridia, cryptorchidism or hypospadias, and hemihypertrophy; it can present with Beckwith-Wiedemann syndrome, a syndrome that consists of exomphalos (congenital umbilical hernia), macroglossia, and gigantism. Wilms' tumor is often associated with neonatal hypoglycemia, ear lobe anomalies, and flame nevus of the face; it is an autosomal recessive inheritance. Wilms' tumor is also present as part of the WAGR syndrome (Wilms' tumor, aniridia, genitourinary malformations, and mental retardation) and Drash's syndrome (male infants with pseudohermaphroditism, Wilms' tumor, mental retardation, and degenerative renal disease). The incidence of neuroblastoma is also increased in patients with pheochromocytomas, neurofibromatosis, Beckwith-Wiedemann syndrome, and Hirschsprung's disease.

Maternal alcohol ingestion is associated with neuroblastoma and hepatoblastoma.

Maternal phenytoin (Dilantin) ingestion is associated with neuroblastoma.

Maternal oral contraceptive use is associated with hepatoblastoma.

Hepatitis B infection (previous or chronic) has a strong association with hepatocellular carcinoma.

Epidemiology

The vast majority of abdominal masses in infancy and childhood are caused by neuroblastoma, Wilms' tumor, or hepatic tumors.

Neuroblastoma is the most common extracranial solid tumor in children and by far the most commonly diagnosed neoplasm in the first year of life, with an incidence rate of 55.2 of 1 million cases. A twofold drop in incidence occurs between the first and second years and a fivefold drop between the first and fifth years of life. Approximately 550 new cases are reported in the United States annually, with a prevalence rate of 1 of 7,000 to 10,000 live births. Neuroblastoma has been seen in utero, and the fetal hormonal secretion may cause hypertension in the mothers of infants. It also has been estimated then that 1 of 250 stillborns has neuroblastoma in situ.

Wilms' tumor typically presents in healthy preschoolers, with an average age of presentation at 3 to 4 years. It is the most common abdominal malignancy and the most common renal malignancy of childhood. The incidence is 500 new cases reported each year in the United States, or approximately 1 of 15,000 live births. Incidence rates decline steadily with age. The kidneys are involved bilaterally in 6% to 7% of patients. Bilaterality has a higher occurrence in girls, in patients with genitourinary anomalies, and in patients who are of a younger age at diagnosis (aged 25 months at diagnosis vs. 44 months).

Approximately two thirds of all **hepatic tumors** are malignant. Table 10.3 lists the categories and associated information regarding benign hepatic tumors. Hepatic malignancies are the tenth most common pediatric cancer. Most are either hepato-

T ABLE 10.3. Benign liver tumors in children

Vascular Tumors (most common benign hepatic tumor)
Hepatic hemangiendothelioma
  Occurs primarily in infants <6 mo of age
  Often associated with cutaneous hemangiomas
  Associated with mass effect, high-output congestive heart failure, bruits, thrombocytopenia
Cavernous hemangioma
  More appropriately designated venous malformation
  Occurs in older children, younger adults
  Usually asymptomatic—can cause congestive heart failure if large
Mesenchymal hamartoma
  Second most common benign hepatic tumor
  Not true neoplasm—developmental anomaly of periportal mesenchyme
  Identified in children <2 y
  Symptoms secondary to mass effect (abdominal distension, respiratory distress)
Hepatic adenoma
  Rare, benign; more common in teenage girls
  Associated with use of oral contraceptives, androgenic steroids
  Associated with type I glycogen storage disease
  50% have abdominal pain, 25% have bleeding from adenoma
Focal nodular hyperplasia
  May occur in response to injury and regeneration
  Asymptomatic
Cysts
  Simple
  Congenital
  3 female: 1 male; whites > blacks
Polycystic
  Inherited
  50% concordance with polycystic kidney disease

blastoma, with an incidence rate of 0.9 of 1 million children, or hepatocellular carcinoma, with an incidence rate of 0.7 of 1 million children. Hepatoblastoma occurs more often in boys, and more than half are diagnosed before the age of 2.

Hepatocullular carcinoma comprises 0.5% to 2% of all pediatric tumors and occurs primarily in adolescents. Hepatocellular carcinoma in the first decade of life has been reported with congenital exposure to hepatitis B.

PATHOPHYSIOLOGY

In **neuroblastoma** is seen malignant growth of the precursors of the sympathetic nervous system. The sympathetic nervous system is derived from the neural crest that provides tissue found in the brain, adrenal medulla, pelvis, mediastinum, and sympathetic ganglia. The oncogenesis of neuroblastoma can be explained by nonrandom chromosomal deletions on chromosome 1, suggesting an absence of a tumor suppressor gene and amplifications of two oncogenes (N-*myc* and N-*ras*).This theory can apply to most neuroblastomas, but some localized tumors do not show this pattern and would suggest another process.

Wilms' tumor originates from renal tissue; histologically, it can be blastemal, stromal, epithelial, or a mixture of these three cell types. One hypothesis suggests a two-staged mutational model proposing that certain deletions in the short arm of chromosome 11 are associated with Wilms' tumor. These deletions are thought to be tumor suppressor genes. These deletions also may support the association with Wilms' tumor and aniridia, and Beckwith-Wiedemann syndrome.

Hepatoblastomas are derived from primitive epithelial parenchyma and result in a lobulated bulging mass originating from the right lobe of the liver. The cause is unknown but one hypothesis suggests a relationship to trisomy 2 and a loss of heterozygosity at chromosome 11.

DIFFERENTIAL DIAGNOSIS

Table 10.4 lists the differential diagnosis for abdominal masses. Abdominal masses in children are caused by an extensive variety of entities. Because abdominal neoplasms most frequently present as an asymptomatic abdominal mass, this chapter focuses on this presentation. A study of the causes of abdominal masses found that 57% were caused by organomegaly. In the other 43%, half involved the urinary tract; the rest were nonrenal and were more likely to be malignant. Research found that multicystic kidney and hydronephrosis were the most common palpable abdominal mass, followed by neuroblastoma and Wilms' tumor. A thorough history, including a review of other presenting symptoms (e.g., pain, weight loss, fever, intestinal obstruction, dysuria, hematuria, melena, jaundice, and duration of symptoms) helps to differentiate among the possibilities. A physical examination can characterize the position, size, surface, configuration, consistency, tenderness, and mobility of the mass. The abdominal quadrant wherein the mass originates provides useful information in making a diagnosis. Masses must be palpated cautiously, especially in the case of a Wilms' tumor where minor trauma can lead to rupture of the mass. Thus far, neuroblastoma, Wilms' tumor, and hepatic neoplasms have been discussed; discussion of other diagnosis in the differential follows.

Other Neoplasms

Rhabdomyosarcoma is a soft tissue sarcoma that usually presents as a lower abdominal painful mass with urinary obstruction. Rhabdomyosarcomas arise in the trigone of the bladder, seminal vesicles, spermatic cord, prostate, vagina, or uterus.

Lymphomas uncommonly present solely with abdominal masses. Associated symptoms include lymphadenopathy, fevers, abdominal pain, abdominal distension, change in bowel habits, nausea and vomiting, early satiety, and blood dyscrasias. Of pediatric patients with non-Hodgkin's lymphoma, 30% to 40% present with abdominal tumors.

Pheochromocytomas are rare tumors that originate from the adrenal medulla. Patients usually have symptoms related to the catecholamine that is secreted from the tumor (i.e., hypertension, sweating, palpitations, tremor, anxiety, headaches, chest and abdominal pain, and electrolyte abnormalities). A family history of pheochromocytomas is frequently elicited.

Mesoblastic nephroma is a congenital renal tumor generally thought to be benign. It presents in infants aged less than 3 months. The tumor is a massive, solitary renal mass, grossly resembling a leiomyoma.

T ABLE 10.14.   Differential diagnosis of abdominal masses

NEOPLASIA
Neuroblastoma
Wilms' tumor
Hepatic tumors
Rhabdomyosarcoma
Lymphoma
Pheochromocytomas
Mesoblastic nephroma
Teratoma

LIVER AND BILIARY DISEASE
Storage diseases (Tay-Sachs, Gaucher, glycogen storage, mucopolysaccharidoses, Niemann-Pick)
Choledochal cyst
Hydrops of the gallbladder
Hepatomegaly from metastasis (leukemia, lymphoma, Wilms' tumor)

GENITOURINARY DISEASE
Polycystic kidney disease
Solitary cysts
Hydronephrosis
Renal vein thrombosis
Ectopic or horseshoe kidney
Ureterocele
Bladder distension
Urachal cyst
Ovarian cyst/tumor
Ovarian torsion
Pregnancy

INTESTINAL DISORDERS
Pyloric stenosis
Intussusception
Fecal material
Volvulus
Bezoar
Intestinal duplication
Incarcerated hernia
Intestinal tumors

MISCELLANEOUS CAUSES
Pancreatic cysts
Abscesses
Peritoneal, mesenteric or omental cysts
Anterior meningocele

Ovarian teratomas are divided into benign and mature cystic teratomas. Most ovarian tumors are benign teratomas. The most common symptoms are nausea and vomiting and pain, although many patients are asymptomatic with abdominal masses noted incidentally.

Liver and Biliary Disorders

Storage diseases (Tay-Sachs, Gaucher, glycogen storage, Niemann-Pick, and mucopolysaccharidoses). Signs and symptoms found on the history and physical examination usually direct the diagnosis (e.g., encephalopathy and other neurologic problems, skeletal abnormalities, visual deterioration, and weight loss).

Choledochol cysts, which can appear as an abdominal mass, are congenital lesions that usually present during the first decade. Usually is seen a classic triad of abdominal pain, jaundice, and mass. Symptoms of acute cholangitis, such as fever, jaundice, and abdominal pain may also be present.

Hydrops of the gallbladder is an acute, noncalculous, noninflammatory distension of the gallbladder that occurs in infants and children. The disorder may complicate acute infections such as scarlet fever or Kawasaki disease. Affected patients usually have right upper quadrant pain and a palpable mass.

Benign hepatic tumors can be diagnosed by a combination of ultrasound, CT, or MRI. Local nodular hyperplasia and mesenchymal hamartoma may require biopsy to distinguish them from malignant lesions.

Genitourinary Disorders

Polycystic kidney disease is the most common hereditary cause of renal cysts. The kidneys are enlarged with multiple small cysts. On physical examination, enlarged kidneys can be mistaken for an abdominal tumor. Symptomatic patients may present with flank pain, hematuria, hypertension, and kidney failure.

Renal cysts are a rare cause of renal mass. They are believed to be retention cysts caused by obstruction of renal tubules.

Renal vein thrombosis is a vascular cause of renal enlargement. It can present as a palpable mass in infancy. Symptoms include a mass, hematuria, and thrombocytopenia. Predisposing factors (i.e. sepsis, congenital heart disease, maternal diabetes) will cause hemoconcentration and thrombosis.

Urachal cysts are remnants of the urachus. They present asymptomatically as a lower midline abdominal mass.

Ovarian tumors will present with varying symptoms depending on whether they are benign or malignant. The symptoms are usually referable to the female genital tract and abdomen, with lower abdominal pain, abdominal mass, and vaginal bleeding being common complaints.

Ovarian torsion presents with pain. A mass may be palpable in the lower quadrants of the abdomen.

Intestinal Disorders

Pyloric stenosis can be diagnosed by palpating a small pyloric mass described as an "olive" in the left upper quadrant of the abdomen. It is usually associated with projectile vomiting in infants aged between 2 and 8 weeks.

Intussusception presents with an abdominal mass in the right upper or lower quadrant. Other symptoms are crampy abdominal pain, lethargy, vomiting, and bloody "currant jelly" stool.

Volvulus should be suspected in children with bilious vomiting and abdominal pain with fullness in the right upper quadrant. Volvulus is a complication of malrotation of the intestine and can lead to necrosis of the midgut around its vascular pedicle. It typically occurs during infancy.

Intestinal duplication is the most common gastrointestinal mass of the newborn. Ileal duplications are the most common, followed by esophageal and colonic. Symptoms usually develop in infancy, although the patient may remain asymptomatic throughout life. Abdominal mass, pain, and distension may be presenting symptoms. Intestinal obstruction can be a complication on intestinal duplications.

Intestinal tumors, which are rare, include carcinoma secondary to ulcerative colitis, lymphoma, and familial polyposis.

Abscesses can occur anywhere in the abdomen. One common cause of abdominal mass in older children is appendiceal abscess. The symptoms are fever, anorexia, nausea, and vomiting, with pain in the right lower quadrant.

Mesenteric or omental cysts can cause abdominal masses. Symptoms of mesenteric cysts consist of a pulling sensation in the abdomen, abdominal distension, and, occasionally, intestinal obstruction. These cysts are secondary to obstruction of the lymphatics. Omental cysts usually are asymptomatic.

REFERRAL

Referral to a pediatric surgeon and pediatric oncologist should be obtained when the initial workup suggests an abdominal tumor. Consultation is required if the diagnosis is unclear.

MANAGEMENT

Management depends on the underlying cause of the abdominal mass. Most patients with abdominal tumors will benefit from consultation with a pediatric oncologist, pediatric surgeon, or both for evaluation and treatment of an abdominal mass.

Neuroblastoma management depends on accurate staging of the tumor. Several staging systems are used for neuroblastoma. They include the Evans classification used by the Pediatric Oncology Group (POG), and the International System for Staging Neuroblastoma (INSS). In the future, the INSS will probably be the standard. Therapy is based on stage, age, tumor size, the presence or absence of metastatic spread, and favorable versus unfavorable prognostic indicators. A tremendous variation is seen in the selection of therapy and new research being done in immunotherapy, adoptive therapy, and gene therapy. Treatment ranges from stage I candidates receiving surgery alone; stage II having surgery and postoperative chemotherapy; and stage III and IV receiving induction chemotherapy, radiation therapy and surgery with follow-up radiation or chemotherapy, radiation with bone marrow ablation, and transplantation. Many complications can occur with aggressive therapy but an aggressive approach increases the chances of survival. Accurate outcome data are difficult to determine, but approximate survival rates are stage I, 100%; stage II, 80%; stage III, 40%; stage IV, 10%; and stage IVs, 80%. This does not factor in other risk factors (e.g., age, where 75% of patients younger than 1 year will survive versus 70% of older patients who will die). New therapies are being designed for all ages and stages.

In **Wilms' tumor,** the National Wilms' Tumor Study group has designed a common staging system that has allowed great advances in treatment. The staging system is shown in Table 10.5. The treatment of Wilms' tumor is complete surgical excision of the entire kidney, ureter, and attached adrenal gland. Currently, all patients receive chemotherapy. However, stage I tumors can be treated with surgery alone with no change in outcome. Radiation therapy is added to stage III and IV disease in patients with favorable histology. The 4-year survival rate for patients with a favorable histology is stage I, 97%; stage II, 95%; stage III, 88%; and stage IV, 82%.

T ABLE 10.5. National Wilms' Tumor Study Group Staging criteria

Stage	Criteria
I	Tumor limited to kidney and completely excised (no spill/no residual tumor)
II	Tumor extends beyond the kidney but is completely removed.
III	Residual *nonhematogeneous* tumor confined to abdomen (lymph nodes, diffuse peritoneal contamination, peritoneal implants).
IV	Hematogeneous metastases (lung, liver, bone and brain).
V	Bilateral renal involvement at diagnosis.

Several modalities are used to treat hepatic neoplasms. Only complete surgical excision can achieve a cure. Preoperative induction chemotherapy may shrink hepatic tumors and allow an unresectable tumor to become resectable. Postoperative chemotherapy is usually needed.

Other Neoplasms

In **rhabdomyosarcoma**, a combination of surgical removal, radiation therapy, and systemic chemotherapy is used.

In **lymphoma**, the primary therapy modality is chemotherapy with surgery and radiation therapy playing secondary roles

In **pheochromocytoma**, therapy with adrenergic antagonists should be initiated to reduce symptoms as well as to prepare for surgical removal of the tumor. The prognosis after successful surgery is excellent.

In **mesoblastic nephroma**, management should be surgical resection.

Liver and Biliary Disorders

Storage diseases, once diagnosed, have different treatments. Some of them can be treated by following specific diets and/or taking supplements to replace the missing enzymes.

Choledochal cysts treatment is primary excision with a Roux-en-Y choledochojejunostomy.

Hydrops of the gallbladder requires treatment of the associated condition (e.g., sepsis, dehydration, Kawasaki disease). Needle or tube cystostomy is rarely required and cholecystectomy is seldom indicated.

Benign hepatic tumors can be observed by serial ultrasounds if small but require resection if they increase in size. Mesenchymal hamartoma and infantile hemangioendothelioma can cause congestive heart failure symptoms that need to be treated with medications.

Genitourinary Disorders

Polycystic kidney disease treatment requires close monitoring (usually by ultrasound) and management of the complications of renal insufficiency. Genetic counseling should also be available.

Treatment of **ovarian tumors** is surgical removal. Recurrences are unusual.

Intestinal Disorders

Pyloric stenosis treatment consists of a pyloromyotomy. This surgical procedure consists of an incision along the pyloric length. It is also important to correct dehydration and other electrolyte abnormalities that may have resulted from preoperative vomiting.

Intussusception may be cured by the diagnostic procedure, the barium enema. If the enema is unsuccessful or if contraindications are seen, surgery is required.

FOLLOW-UP

Patients with neuroblastoma, Wilms' tumor, and hepatic neoplasms need to be closely followed by a pediatric oncologist. All patients with recurrences have a poorer prognosis.

PATIENT EDUCATION

Because most patients who present with abdominal tumors are asymptomatic, it is important to instruct parents that if they notice a mass or if the abdominal girth increases, they should notify their family physician immediately. The prognoses of all abdominal neoplasms are improved the earlier they are found. In addition, patients with certain conditions that are associated with abdominal tumors (e.g., Beckwith-Wiedemann syndrome, aniridia, cryptorchidism) should be followed closely to assess for any abdominal masses.

SUGGESTED READING

Castleberry RP. Biology and treatment of neuroblastoma. *Pediatr Clin North Am* 1997;44:919-937.

Caty MG, Shamberger RC. Abdominal tumors in infancy and childhood. *Pediatr Clin North Am* 1993;40:1253-1271.

Gurney JG, Severson RK, Davis S, et al. Incidence of cancer in children in the United States. Sex, race, and 1-year age-specific rates by histologic types. *Cancer* 1995;75: 2186-2195.

Pearl R, Irish M, Caty M, Glick PL. The approach to common abdominal diagnoses in infants and children. Pediatric surgery for the primary care physician. Part II. *Pediatr Clin North Am* 1998;45:1-35.

Pizzo PA, Horowitz ME, Poplack DG, et al. Solid tumors of childhood. In: Devita JT Jr., Hellman S, Rosenberg SA, eds. *Cancer: principles and practice of oncology*, 3rd ed. Philadelphia: JB Lippincott; 1989:1612.

Steuber CP, Nesbit ME. Clinical assessment and differential diagnosis of the child with suspected cancers. In: Pizzo PA, Poplack DC, eds. *Principles and practice of pediatric oncology*, 3rd ed. Philadelphia: Lippincott-Raven; 1997:129.

Warner BW. Consultation with the specialist—Wilms' tumor. *Pediatr Rev* 1996;17: 371-373.

CHAPTER 11

Constipation

Jory A. Natkin and Martin S. Lipsky

DEFINITION

Constipation is a common medical problem, accounting for more than 2.5 million physician visits in the United States annually. Despite its prevalence, no uniform definition of constipation is found. Although stool habits vary significantly with age, diet, and geography, population studies suggest most normal persons eating an average Western diet will pass at least three stools per week. Therefore, one objective and clinically useful definition is the passage of fewer than three stools per week.

CLINICAL MANIFESTATIONS

The clinical manifestations of constipation vary widely. Patients can experience a sense of incomplete evacuation, straining, and passing hard, lumpy stools, as well as a decrease in stool frequency. Individuals may also complain of feeling bloated and gassy and experience abdominal discomfort. In addition to a decreased number of bowel movements, patients may have signs and symptoms associated with an underlying problem. For example, weight loss and anemia combined with constipation could herald the presence of an underlying colon cancer. Alternating constipation with diarrhea in an otherwise healthy patient is a classic symptom of irritable bowel syndrome. Patients with anorectal disease complain of painful defecation.

PATIENT HISTORY

The patient history is useful in determining the underlying cause of constipation. Eliciting the chronicity, character, and severity of associated complaints is important. Because of such a wide range of what is considered normal stool frequency, many patients may not be experiencing true constipation.

Chronic constipation, without a recent change in bowel habits, is far more likely to be a functional problem. Inquiring about diet, hydration, and activity is important. Patients with low dietary fiber intake usually have intermittent complaints that resolve with diet alteration. Constipation is common in patients who lead a sedentary lifestyle or in active people who decrease their activity level, either voluntarily or because of illness.

It is important to inquire about medication use because drugs can have an important impact on bowel habits. Opiates and anticholinergic agents (e.g., tricyclic antidepressants) are common causes of drug-induced constipation. Calcium channel agents can decrease gastrointestinal mobility and antacids containing aluminum or calcium can also cause constipation. Habitual use of laxatives can sometimes damage the colon and impair motility and lead to constipation. Drugs associated with constipation are listed in Table 11.1.

T ABLE 11.1. Drugs associated with constipation

Analgesics

Anticholinergics
Antispasmodics
Antidepressants
Antipsychotics
Antiparkinsonian drugs

Cation-Containing Agents
Iron supplements
Aluminum (antacids, sucralfate)
Calcium (antacids, supplements)
Barium sulfate
Metallic intoxication (arsenic, lead, mercury)

Neurally Active Agents
Opiates
Antihypertensives
Ganglionic blockers
Vinca alkaloids
Anticonvulsants
Calcium channel blockers

From Wald A. Approach to the patient with constipation. In: Yamada T, Alpers DH, Laine L, Owyang C, Powell DW, eds. *Textbook of gastroenterology*, 3rd ed. Philadelphia: Lippincott Williams & Wilkins, 1999:911; with permission.

Constipation with abdominal pain can indicate a variety of conditions (e.g., tumor, stricture, or volvulus). Rectal bleeding or new onset constipation in an older individual increases the likelihood of colonic cancer. Rectal pain with defecation suggests an anal or perianal condition, such as a thrombosed hemorrhoid, fissure, or rectal abscess.

The history can provide clues that suggest a metabolic, endocrine, or neurologic disease. Hypokalemia can produce an ileus and is most often seen in conjunction with diuretic therapy. Symptoms such as fatigue and cold intolerance suggest hypothyroidism. Disorders causing significant hypercalcemia can also lead to constipation. Diabetic individuals with evidence of a neuropathy frequently experience constipation.

Neurologic impairment sometimes presents with constipation. The history may elicit symptoms suggestive of Parkinson's disease or multiple sclerosis. A history of constipation because infancy raises the possibility of defective colonic motility, such as seen in Hirschsprung's disease. Table 11.2 lists characteristic features that help differentiate a functional disorder from colon neuromuscular disorders such as Hirschsprung's disease in children. Discussing bowel habits also helps identify individuals who fail to allow adequate time for defecation or repeatedly ignore the urge to defecate. Both of these practices can lead to constipation.

T ABLE 11.2. Features of functional versus neuromuscular disorders in children

Characteristic	Functional	Neuromuscular
Fecal soiling	Common	Rare
Large-caliber stools	Common	Rare
Stool withholding	Common	Rare
Upper gastrointestinal symptoms	Rare	Common
Symptoms from birth	Rare	Common
Localization of stools	Rectum	Colon and rectum

PHYSICAL EXAMINATION

The physical examination is useful for identifying potential causes and guiding the diagnostic workup.

Check the abdomen for masses, distention tenderness, and bowel sounds. A distended abdomen with decreased bowel sounds and stool in the rectal vault is consistent with an ileus. In contrast, distention, high-pitched bowel sounds, and an empty vault suggest obstruction. Palpation of a mass suggests the possibility of a neoplasm. Abdominal tenderness without a mass is characteristic of irritable bowel syndrome.

A careful rectal examination is important for detecting an impaction, rectal mass, fissure, abscess, or rectal bleeding. Also look for underlying nongastrointestinal disease. Neurologic findings (e.g., tremor or rigidity), particularly in older individual, raise the possibility of Parkinson's disease. Orthostatic changes and diminished reflexes may suggest a neuropathy. Dry skin and diminished reflexes are consistent with hypothyroidism. A pelvic examination is important for detecting mass lesions in women.

DIAGNOSTIC STUDIES

The use of diagnostic testing to determine the cause of a patient's constipation depends on the history and physical findings. Patients with acute onset constipation or chronic constipation with a recent change may benefit from a laboratory evaluation. Useful tests include a complete blood cell count to detect anemia and a chemical profile to exclude metabolic disorders such as hypokalemia, hypercalcemia, and diabetes. A thyroid-stimulating hormone test is also useful to exclude hypothyroidism.

Anoscopy and sigmoidoscopy can detect pathology of the anus, rectum, and sigmoid colon. Anoscopy may reveal fissures, hemorrhoids, or a mass. Flexible sigmoidoscopy can help rule out an obstructive lesion or identify the brownish mucosal discoloration seen in melanosis coli. In patients with constipation since childhood, a submucosal rectal biopsy can diagnose Hirschsprung's disease by demonstrating the absence of neurons. Biopsy findings of melanosis coli suggest chronic laxative abuse. A colonoscopy is indicated in cases of suspected malignancy.

Radiographic procedures are of limited value unless the history and physical examination findings suggest a specific cause such as obstruction. An abdominal series can be useful for detecting acute obstruction, or revealing gas patterns consistent with an ileus, Hirschsprung's disease, or a volvulus. Abdominal films also provide information about the amount and distribution of stool.

Rarely, colonic transit studies may be useful in patients whose only complaint is infrequent stooling. In these studies, patients ingest radio opaque markers. Serial radiographs monitor transit through the colon. Delayed transit times indicate a physiologic cause, whereas normal times suggest a psychological or behavioral cause. Holdup of markers in the rectal vault reflects an outlet problem in contrast to the even distribution of markers throughout the colon and rectum seen in colonic inertia.

Patients with constipation recalcitrant to treatment or those who require large doses of laxatives may benefit from specialized testing such as anorectal manometry or defecography. Rectal manometry supplies information about sphincter function and rectal sensation, and is useful to rule out Hirschsprung's disease. Defecography may be useful in patients who complain of straining during defecation. It provides information about completeness of evacuation and musculature and anatomic abnormalities (e.g., a rectocele).

RISK FACTORS

Risk factors for constipation include the aforementioned underlying diseases—hypothyroidism, hyperparathyroidism, and diabetes. Neurologic disorders, such as stroke, Parkinson's disease, multiple sclerosis, and spinal cord injuries, are also significant risk factors for constipation.

Inadequate dietary fiber intake, poor fluid intake, and psychological disorders can be contributing factors. Laxative abuse, more common in women than men, is also associated with constipation. Polypharmacy, which can result in individuals taking more than one potentially constipating agent, is also a risk factor.

Lifestyle factors can also place individuals at risk. Sedentary lifestyle, nursing home residence, or an illness that causes inactivity can also cause constipation. A hectic lifestyle that precludes allowing sufficient time for defecation also places patients at risk.

PATHOPHYSIOLOGY

Defecation depends on a normal stool volume to adequately stimulate the colon, normal intestinal motility, normal sensory function to perceive the presence of stool, and normal stool consistency to facilitate rectal emptying. Actual defecation requires a complex interaction between the central nervous system and the muscles that increase intraabdominal pressure, relax the sphincter, and open the anal canal.

The gastrocolic reflex is colonic stimulation following ingestion of a meal. Repeated suppression can lead to constipation. Normal colonic motility is impaired by physical inactivity. A low-fiber diet or inadequate fluid intake decreases stool volume and consistency and can lead to constipation. Neuromuscular diseases, such as Hirschsprung's disease, multiple sclerosis, spinal cord injury, and diabetes can also alter colon mobility.

Anorectal disorders (e.g., fissures or thrombosed hemorrhoids) that cause pain can lead to constipation by causing avoidance of defecation. Mechanical obstruction, such as seen in cancer stricture or external compression, is another pathophysiologic mechanism for constipation.

DIFFERENTIAL DIAGNOSIS

Table 11.3 lists the extensive differential diagnosis for constipation. The history and physical examination findings frequently suggest whether constipation is the result of a structural abnormality, diet, medication side effect, metabolic disease, or a neu-

TABLE 11.3. Differential diagnosis for constipation

ENVIRONMENTAL/BEHAVIORAL
Inadequate fiber/fluid intake
Reduced physical activity
Psychologic factors

DRUG SIDE EFFECTS

METABOLIC/ENDOCRINE/SYSTEMIC DISEASE
Hypothyroidism
Adrenal insufficiency
Hypercalcemia
Hyperparathyroidism
Diabetes mellitus
Uremia
Hypomagnesemia

NEUROMUSCULAR
Intestinal myopathy
Intestinal neuropathy
Cerebrovascular accident
Spinal cord injury
Multiple sclerosis
Parkinson's disease
Autonomic dysfunction
Amyotrophic lateral sclerosis
Hirschsprung's disease
Amyloidosis
Scleroderma
Chagas' disease

ANATOMIC CONDITIONS
Gastrointestinal tumors
Strictures
Pregnancy
Pelvic tumors/masses
Anorectal disease (fissures, fistulas, masses)
External compression of the intestine
Adhesion
Colonic volvulus
Intussusception
Hernia

OTHER CONDITIONS
Depression
Dementia
Immobility
Cardiac disease
Irritable bowel syndrome

romuscular disorder. The acuity of onset and the degree of suspicion that an associated disorder is present should direct the evaluation. For example, in a younger patient whose clinical evaluation indicates a benign cause (e.g., a drug side effect or insufficient fiber), management may be initiated. Those who respond to treatment need no further evaluation. Conversely, an older patient with an acute onset of constipation and associated symptoms (e.g., Hemoccult-positive stool, weight loss, and anemia) merits colonoscopy.

In refractory cases or in cases where the cause is uncertain, laboratory testing may be helpful. A typical workup includes testing stools for occult blood and a complete blood cell count to detect anemia. Chemical profile screens for metabolic causes and a serum thyroid-stimulating hormone test assesses thyroid function.

A barium enema or colonoscopy can evaluate structural lesions. The presence of a dilated colon or rectal biopsy can rule in Hirschsprung's disease.

REFERRAL

Referral to a gastroenterologist may be necessary when colonoscopy is appropriate. Difficult cases with or those without a diagnosis after workup by the family physician may need input by a specialist. Structural lesions or neoplasms need surgical evaluation. Persistent constipation also merits referral to a gastroenterologist for specialized studies, such as anorectal manometry and defecography. In some geographic areas, these specialized tests are difficult to arrange and may be available only at a tertiary care hospital.

MANAGEMENT

The treatment of constipation depends on the underlying cause. It can include hormone replacement for hypothyroidism or hospitalization and surgery for the patient with an obstruction.

Discontinue any nonessential medication associated with causing constipation. Often this will resolve the problem.

Dietary changes are also crucial for treating constipation. Decreasing refined carbohydrates, adequate fluid intake, exercise, and maximizing soluble dietary fiber may be all that is needed to treat most constipated patients. The minimal amount of dietary fiber should range from 10 to 20 g/d. Table 11.4 lists food sources of dietary fiber. Nearly all patients experience temporary bloating, gas, and cramping during the first few weeks of fiber supplementation. Warn patients of these side effects and recommend that they increase the amount of fiber slowly. For example, if a supplement such as psyllium is used, a typical regimen might be to start with 1 tsp daily, then increase the dose at weekly intervals (by 1 tsp/d) until constipation resolves or a maximum dose is reached. It is essential that patients maintain adequate fluid intake when using bulk laxatives such as psyllium. Otherwise, these agents can exacerbate constipation. The chronic use of laxatives should be strongly discouraged because, as mentioned, they are a common cause of constipation. Most patients can eventually stop all other laxatives when a high-fiber diet and sufficient fluid intake are initiated.

Osmotic laxatives, such as lactulose or Milk of Magnesia, work by increasing the water content of the stool. These laxatives have the advantage of not causing damage to the colon when used over a long period of time. In patients who do not respond to fiber or who cannot tolerate bulking agents, osmotic agents (e.g., lactulose or sorbitol) are the preparations of choice. Magnesium-containing compounds should be avoided in patients with renal insufficiency. When used, start with a mild laxative, such as magnesium hydroxide (Milk of Magnesia). Magnesium sulfate and magnesium citrate are more potent.

T ABLE 11.4. Food sources of dietary fiber

	Amount of serving (g)	Amount/100 g of food
Breakfast Cereals		
All-Bran	9.9	26.70
Cornflakes	2.8	11.00
Rice Krispies	1.4	4.51
Shredded Wheat	3.0	12.31
Special K	1.7	5.41
Breads		
White bread	0.8	2.71
Whole wheat	2.4	8.51
Fruits		
Apple	3.2	1.41
Banana	5.9	1.71
Peach	2.1	2.38
Pear	3.1	2.41
Strawberry	3.3	2.12
Nuts		
Brazil	5.4	7.71
Peanut	5.7	9.31
Peanut butter	2.1	7.51
Vegetables		
Broccoli	5.6	4.11
Cabbage	1.9	2.81
Cauliflower	2.5	1.81
Lettuce	0.8	1.51
Carrot	3.7	3.20
Baked beans	18.6	7.31
Peas	11.3	6.31
Tomato	3.0	1.41

From Yang P, Banwell JG. Dietary fiber: its role in the pathogenesis and treatment of constipation. *Pract Gastroenterol* 1986;10:28.

If mild laxatives are ineffective, stimulant laxatives (e.g., bisacodyl or senna) are the typical next choices. These laxatives are to be used for refractory symptoms and only on an as-needed basis. Suppositories and enemas can also be used for treatment when a prompt result is desired. Although widely used, stool softeners are generally not effective. Table 11.5 lists some common medications used for constipation. All these agents have the potential to induce diarrhea. In cases when constipation is severe, it may be helpful to use intensive initial therapy, such as a nonabsorbed bowel preparation (e.g., GoLytely, Colyte, Miralax) to cleanse the colon, followed by the

T ABLE 11.5. Medications for constipation

Medications	Side effects
Bulk Agents	
Psyllium (Metamucil), 1 tablespoon qd–tid	Bloating, impaction above strictures
Methycellulose (Citrucel), 1–3 tablespoons qd	Fluid overload, impaction with insufficient fluid
Calcium polycarbophil (Fibercon), 1 tablet qd–tid	Fluid overload, impaction
Softeners	
Dioctyl sodium (Colace), 1–2 capsules qd	Skin rashes, hepatotoxicity
Stimulants	
Bisacodyl (Dulcolax), 1–2 tablets or suppositories qd	Gastric or rectal irritation
Senna (Senokot), 1–3 teaspoons, 2–3 tablets qd	Degeneration of myoneural plexuses
Casanthranol (Peri-Colace), 1–2 tablets qd	Degeneration of myoneural plexuses
Osmotics	
Lactulose (Cephulac), 1–2 tablespoons qd	Bloating
Magnesium (Milk of Magnesia, Magnesium citrate)	Magnesium toxicity (with renal failure)
Sorbitol 70%, 2–4 tablespoons qd	Bloating

qd, every day; qhs, every night; tid, three times daily.

Modified from Wald A. Approach to the patient with constipation. In: Yamada T, Alpers DH, Laine L, Owyang C, Powell DW, eds. *Textbook of Gastroenterology*, 3rd ed. Philadelphia: Lippincott Williams & Wilkins; 1999:921.

addition of fiber or laxatives in a stepwise fashion as needed to achieve a reasonable frequency and consistency of stool.

FOLLOW-UP

Patients with an underlying disease causing constipation always need to be monitored. It is also necessary to monitor response to dietary changes. Ask about bowel habits, including bowel movement frequency, consistency, and any straining or pain associated with them. Stress in the patient's daily life at home and work is an important factor that also needs to be followed.

Other complications of constipation include fecal impaction, increased urinary tract infections in women, and a theoretical increase in colorectal carcinoma. Patients with chronic constipation, particularly in settings such as long-term care facilities, need to be monitored for fecal impaction.

PATIENT EDUCATION

Many patients have misconceptions about what normal bowel habits should be. The physician or other healthcare professional needs to educate patients about the facts of healthy bowel habits and what they can do on their own to treat and avoid constipation. Avoiding long-term laxative use is important. Patients need a detailed explanation why, after long-term use, a laxative is being stopped. It is important to tell chronic laxative users that it can take 4 to 6 weeks before their bowel movements normalize. Patience, empathy, and continued support are critical for success whenever a new bowel regimen is started.

Also advise patients that constipation might be a side effect of certain medications, such as narcotic pain relievers. Bowel retraining may be needed when the cause is functional or no cause of the patient's complaint has been identified. In addition, instruct patients about other lifestyle changes (e.g., increased physical activity), which may be beneficial in treating and preventing further constipation.

SUGGESTED READING

Enomoto KD, Yen YET. Constipation. In: Taylor RB, ed. *Manual of family practice.* Boston: Little, Brown & Co.; 1997.

Felt B, Wise C, Olson A, Kochhar P, Marcus S, Coran A. Guideline for the management of pediatric idiopathic constipation and soiling. *Arch Pediatr Adolesc Med* 1999; 153:380-385.

Frank D. Constipation. In: Dambro MR, ed. *Griffith's 5-minute clinical consult.* Philadelphia: Lippincott Williams & Wilkins; 2000.

Schaefer DC, Cheskin LJ. Constipation in the elderly. *Am Fam Physician* 1998;58: 907-914.

Yamada T. Approach to the patient with constipation. In: Yamada T, ed. *Handbook of gastroenterology.* Philadelphia: Lippincott Williams & Wilkins; 1998.

CHAPTER 12

Acute Diarrhea

Martin S. Lipsky

DEFINITION

Diarrhea is one of the most common conditions encountered in family practice. Acute diarrhea is defined as the passage of abnormally loose stools, usually associated with excessive frequency of defecation (> 3 per 24 hours) that lasts less than 2 weeks.

CLINICAL MANIFESTATIONS

Acute diarrhea can usually be divided into two clinical presentations: (a) a watery noninflammatory diarrhea, or (b) an inflammatory diarrhea with a presence of either blood or white blood cells. The history is important for assessing the severity of illness and for classifying the illness into one of these two categories. From the standpoint of severity, diarrhea can be categorized as being mild, with no change in normal activity; moderate, with some forced limitation in activity; or severe, where patients are confined to bed.

In patients with acute diarrhea, ask about any recent travel, exposure to others with similar symptoms, recent antibiotic or other medication use, recent illnesses, and their diets. Laxative abuse, excessive caffeine or alcohol intake, and sorbitol-containing foods can all cause transient diarrhea.

Antibiotic therapy within 2 weeks of the onset of diarrhea suggests either an alteration of bowel flora or *Clostridium difficile* infection. Over-indulgence of milk or milk products in a lactose-intolerant individual can also result in acute symptoms.

Acute infectious diarrheas most commonly present with watery stools. In infants and young children, the most common cause is rotavirus. Rotavirus is often preceded by a brief prodrome with fever and may be accompanied by nausea or vomiting. Typically, the illness lasts about 7 days. Viral diarrhea caused from adenovirus infections is associated with respiratory symptoms and a slightly longer course.

Infectious diarrhea in adults is also usually viral, but is more likely to be bacterial than in children. In travelers, enterotoxigenic *Escherichia coli* infection is a common cause. Toxigenic *E. coli* diarrhea usually begins after a short incubation period and lasts an average of 3 to 5 days. It is associated with nausea, vomiting, abdominal cramps, bloating, and a low grade fever.

Although many invasive pathogens and protozoa illnesses can produce a clinical picture similar to watery diarrhea, invasive pathogens such as *Shigella*, *Salmonella*, and *Campylobacter* more often present with bloody diarrhea. These infections typically have a prodrome with a low-grade fever, headache, anorexia, and lassitude. Stools initially may be watery and then become bloody later in the illness. Lower abdominal cramping is a common feature of a dysenteric illness.

Diarrhea that comes only hours after eating suggests a preformed toxin in contaminated food, particularly if others eating the same food have similar symptoms.

Noninfectious and extraintestinal processes can also present as acute diarrhea in adults. Severe abdominal pain associated with diarrhea in older patients, particularly those with evidence of vascular disease, suggests an ischemic bowel. Inflammatory bowel disease can also present fulminantly as acute diarrhea. Partial bowel obstruction, pelvic abscess, fecal impaction, and diverticulosis can also present as acute diarrhea.

PHYSICAL EXAMINATION

Physical examination is rarely helpful in determining the cause of diarrhea. Fever higher than 38.5°C (101.3°F.) is more common in bacterial illnesses but can be seen in viral syndromes. Orthostatic changes, hypotension, tachycardia, dry mucous membranes, and poor skin turgor suggest significant volume loss. Examine the abdomen for tenderness, masses, and organomegaly. Auscultation may reveal hyperactive bowel sounds with acute infectious diarrhea. A rectal examination is done looking for skin lesions, to confirm the gross appearance of the stool, and to test for occult blood.

RISK FACTORS

Infants, young children, and the elderly are more susceptible to infection. The elderly may be more susceptible because of declining immune function and decreased gastric acid secretion. The acidic stomach environment acts as a physical barrier to infection and a higher pH increases the risk of infection.

Travel outside the United States and Canada, particularly to areas with inadequate sanitation, increases an individual's risk for diarrheal illnesses, most commonly enterotoxigenic *E. coli*. Endemic areas for *Giardia* organisms include the Rocky Mountains, Russia, and Italy.

Hospitalization or antibiotic use within 6 weeks increases the risk of *C. difficile*. Ampicillin, clindamycin, and cephalosporins are among the most common antibiotics associated with *C. difficile*, but nearly all antimicrobial agents have been implicated.

Impaired immunity is a well-recognized risk factor. Table 12.1 lists causes of infectious diarrhea in individuals infected with the human immunodeficiency virus (HIV).

T ABLE 12.1. Common causes of infectious diarrhea in HIV-infected individuals

Protozoa	*Cryptosporidium parvum*
	Microsporium spp
	Giardia
	Isospora belli
	Cyclospora
	Entamoeba histolytica
Bacterial	*Salmonella* spp
	Shigella spp
	Campylobacter spp
	Vibrio parahaemolyticus
	Mycobacterium avium complex
Virus	*Cytomegalovirus*

From Porro GB, ed. *Gastroenterology and Hepatology.* New York: McGraw-Hill; 1999; with permission.

Cryptosporidium spp., *Isospora* spp., and *Mycobacterium avium-intracellulare* most often cause recurrent episodes of acute diarrhea. Cancer chemotherapy is also a risk factor for opportunistic infections, such as cytomegalovirus and *C. difficile.*

Salmonella infections are frequently traced to infected eggs, poultry, or pet turtles. *Campylobacter* infection is linked to the ingestion of raw milk, poultry, and untreated water. Invasive *E. coli* is associated with the ingestion of unpasteurized milk, uncooked ground beef, and contaminated water. Custard-filled pastries, potato salad, egg salad, and processed meats can become contaminated with *Staphylococcus aureus*, which can produce a toxin capable of causing acute diarrhea. *Clostridium perfringens* is another common food-borne contaminate found in poorly reheated meats and in poultry and foods that have been warmed on steam tables.

EPIDEMIOLOGY

Gastrointestinal infections are the most common intestinal disorder. Despite higher levels of sanitation, acute intestinal infections are increasing in the United States. Almost 100 million cases occur annually and acute diarrhea accounts for 1.5% of the hospitalizations for adults and 6.5% of pediatric admissions. Factors contributing to the rise include increased use of broad-spectrum antibiotics, increased number of patients with impaired immunity from HIV or cancer therapy, and an increase in travel to third-world countries.

Infected humans are the major reservoir for bacterial and protozoal infections and may be the only reservoir for enteric viruses. For *Shigella* and amebiasis, humans are the only known reservoir.

PATHOPHYSIOLOGY

Most intestinal pathogens are transmitted through the fecal-oral route. Gastric acid is a prime defense mechanism because many enteric pathogens are sensitive to an acidic environment.

Most enteropathogens attach to the intestinal epithelial cells. Invasive organisms, such as *Shigella, Salmonella*, and *Campylobacter jejuni*, which attach and invade the mucosa lining the bowel wall, can produce invasive inflammatory disease. Although *Entamoeba histolytica* produces inflammation, it is not truly invasive. Instead, after binding to the colon lining, the amoeba produces a potent protein which induces epithelial disruption. The amoeba then phagocytizes the dead epithelium cell and moves deeper into the mucosa.

Rotavirus and other viruses can attach directly to the small intestinal epithelial cells. All these infections can disrupt the intestinal absorptive surface, resulting in diarrhea. Some organisms (e.g., *Vibrio cholera* and enterotoxigenic *E. coli*) produce enterotoxins that stimulate fluid secretions. Other pathogens (e.g., *Shigella, C. difficile*, and invasive *E. coli*) produce substances that are toxic to the epithelial cells.

DIFFERENTIAL DIAGNOSIS

Table 12.2 lists common causes of intestinal infections in infants and children. Other causes of acute diarrhea in children include diarrhea secondary to infections (e.g., a urinary tract infection), medicines, food poisoning, dietary indiscretion, and inflammatory bowel disease.

Most patients with acute diarrhea have mild, self-limiting symptoms, and medical evaluation should be limited to patients with more severe illness. Indications for evaluation include moderate to severe symptoms such as dehydration, more than six stools per 24 hours, symptoms that persist beyond 48 to 72 hours, stools con-

T ABLE 12.2. Causes of infectious diarrhea in infants and children

Viruses	Rotavirus
	Enteric adenovirus (types 40,41)
	Norwalk virus
Bacterial	Enteropathogenic *Escherichia coli*
	Enterotoxigenic *E. coli*
	Salmonella spp
	Shigella spp
	Campylobacter spp
	Yersinia spp
	Aeromontas spp
Protozoa	*Giardia*
	Entamoeba histolytica
	Cryptosporidium

From Porro GB, ed. *Gastroenterology and Hepatology.* New York: McGraw-Hill; 1999; with permission.

taining blood or mucus, temperature higher than 38.5°C (101.3°F), diarrhea associated with severe abdominal pain, and diarrhea in older or immunocompromised patients.

Routine blood tests are generally not helpful in making a specific diagnosis. However, they are useful in detecting electrolyte abnormalities in patients with severe diarrhea. In acute bloody diarrhea an associated anemia or evidence of an inflammatory process, such as an elevated neutrophil count, a raised platelet count, or an elevated erythrocyte sedimentation rate may be found.

Examining stools for fecal leukocytes and occult blood is the first step in evaluating patients with acute diarrhea. These studies distinguish between inflammatory versus noninflammatory causes. To examine the stool for leukocytes, a small amount of fresh stool is diluted with saline and then put on a microscope slide. A few drops of methylene blue are added and a cover slip is placed over the mixture. A finding of more than three or four white blood cells per high-powered field suggests an inflammatory process. Most patients with noninflammatory watery diarrhea have an illness that is self-limited. Further investigation is generally unnecessary.

If an inflammatory process is suspected, either clinically or by white blood cells in the stool, send stool cultures to detect *Salmonella, Shigella, Campylobacter,* and *Aeromonas* organisms. Testing for other enteropathogens, such as *Yersinia, Vibrio,* and pathogenic forms of *E. coli* requires special methods; if these organisms are clinically suspected, the microbiology department should be notified. A stool specimen should be examined for *C. difficile* toxin in patients with recent antibiotic use or hospitalization or in those who reside in a long-term care facility. Noninfectious causes of acute bloody diarrhea include an acute presentation of inflammatory bowel disease, ischemic colitis, diverticular disease, and colonic neoplasm.

Stool examination for ova and parasites is indicated for patients at risk for *Giardia* or other parasitic infections. Because numerous leukocytes are not usually seen in patients with intestinal amebiasis, the diagnosis should be considered in patients with dysentery but few leukocytes present in the stool.

Sigmoidoscopy should be considered for patients with prominent rectal symptoms and culture-negative patients with inflammatory diarrhea.

DIAGNOSTIC STUDIES

Table 12.3 lists diagnostic clues with additional tests that may be useful in determining the diagnosis. Stool cultures will detect the classic enteropathogens, but light microscopy is needed to detect the cysts and trophozoites of *E. histolytica*. If enterotoxigenic *E. coli* is suspected, *E. coli* colonies present in the stool culture must be subcultured and stereotyped. The clinical relevance of a culture that grows *C. difficile* can be confirmed by the presence of *C. difficile* toxin in the stool. In patients with invasive *E. histolytica*, the results of serologic analysis are positive in approximately 80% to 90% of samples, and as such may be useful.

Imaging has a very limited role in acute infectious diarrhea. A common finding on plain abdominal radiographs is multiple small bowel fluid levels and mild small bowel dilatation. A loss of haustra and colonic dilatation is indicative of severe colitis.

Colonoscopy is useful for examining the appearance of the colon and obtaining tissue for histologic examination. Although differentiation between acute infectious colitis and other forms of colitis can be difficult, an experienced endoscopist may be able to identify amoebic ulceration. If *E. histolytica* is suspected, scrapings from ulcerations can be examined for the presence of amoeba. Ischemic colitis can be identified by regional involvement of the splenic flexure or proximal descending colon along with a dark, dusky red mucosa seen during colonoscopy. Colonoscopy can also detect the presence of a pseudomembrane, a pale yellowish plaque on top of reddened, edematous mucosa, which bleeds if removed. These plaques are usually separated by areas of normal mucosa and are generally indicative of *C. difficile* infections. However, they are not specific for *C. difficile* and can occur in other conditions, such as ischemia.

T ABLE 12.3.   Historical diagnostic clues, causes, and relevant tests

Diagnostic clue	Possible cause	Additional test
Bloody stools	*Salmonella, Shigella, Campylobacter,* invasive *Escherichia coli, Clostridium difficile, Entamoeba histolytica,* inflammatory bowel disease, ischemic colitis, neoplasm,	Stool culture, stool for ova, and parasites, *C. difficile* toxin, colonoscopy
Recent hospitalization or antibiotic treatment	*C. difficile,* drugs	Stool for *C. difficile* toxin
Several close contacts with those affected acutely	Food poisoning	None
Severe or persistent abdominal pain	*Campylobacter* spp *Yersinia* spp	Notify laboratory for special culture
Day care center or institutionalized	*Giardia, C. difficile, Salmonella* spp, *Shigella* spp, rotavirus	Stool for *C. difficile* toxin, stool for ova and parasites
Rectal pain, tenesmus	*Campylobacter* spp, *Salmonella* spp, *Shigella* spp, gonococcus, herpes, chlamydia, *E. histolytica,* inflammatory bowel disease	Sigmoidoscopy with cultures, possible biopsy

REFERRAL

Patients with evidence of severe dehydration or marked symptoms must be admitted to the hospital for intravenous fluids, diagnostic workup, and treatment.

Suspected sources of contaminated foods should be reported to the public health department for evaluation. HIV patients with diarrhea and patients with persistent symptoms may respond to empiric treatment. However, prolonged and recurrent symptoms may need referral to a gastroenterologist for evaluation.

MANAGEMENT

Fluid therapy, an alteration in diet, and monitoring for resolution of symptoms are appropriate management steps for most patients with acute diarrhea. Oral rehydration is the first choice for restoring fluid balance. Special attention should be given to infants, young children, and the elderly. Commercial rehydration solutions (e.g., Pedialyte) are designed to replace both fluids and electrolytes. Also available are commercial cereal-based oral rehydration solutions (e.g., Ricelyte). These solutions may offer the advantage of reducing the volume of diarrhea.

Sports drinks, diluted fruit drinks, and flavored soft drinks augmented with crackers, soups, or broth can adequately replace fluids in a mildly dehydrated healthy adult or an older child with acute diarrhea. A younger child or infant is better managed with a commercial rehydration solution or by preparing a rehydration fluid that contains approximately 60 to 90 mEq/L of sodium, 20 mEq/L of potassium, 80 mEq/L of chloride, and 20 g/L of glucose. One example of how to prepare a homemade rehydration solution is to mix 3/4 tsp salt, 1 tsp baking soda, 1 cup orange juice, and 4 tsp sugar in 1 L of clear water. Rehydration solutions are preferable to such commonly recommended clear liquids as apple juice, carbonated beverages, and chicken soup, which do not adequately replace lost electrolytes and can precipitate osmotic diarrhea. A homemade, cereal-based solution can be prepared by mixing 1/2 cup of baby rice cereal with 2 cups of water and 1/4 tsp of salt.

Although vomiting is common in children with acute diarrheal illnesses, most children can still be rehydrated orally by giving small amounts of fluid frequently, such as 5 ml by teaspoon or oral syringe every 5 minutes. The child with mild dehydration needs approximately 50 ml/kg over the first 6 hours, whereas the goal for a child with moderate dehydration is approximately 100 ml/kg. In a formula-fed infant, fluids can consist of alternate feedings of formula and rehydration solution. Table 12.4 outlines fluid therapy in more detail. Vomiting usually ceases as soon as rehydration is underway.

Avoiding milk products and caffeine-containing products can also be helpful. Boiled starches (potatoes, rice, noodles) with some salt are good foods for patients with acute diarrhea. Patients with marked dehydration may need hospitalization for evaluation and treatment.

Although it has been common practice to "rest" the bowel in children with diarrhea, most authorities believe this practice actually prolongs the course of diarrhea. As soon as a child is rehydrated, full-strength formula or breast-feeding can be initiated. Older children can be started on a carbohydrate-rich diet. Although commonly used, no evidence indicates that the traditional BRAT (bananas, rice, apples, toast) diet is beneficial.

The use of antibiotics depends on the organism, the health of the individual, and the presence of systemic symptoms. Choices for antibiotics are summarized in Table 12.5. All patients with confirmed *Shigella* infection should be treated with antibiotics. Trimethoprim combined with sulfamethoxazole (TMP/SMZ; Bactrim) is an acceptable therapy for *Shigella* infections acquired in the United States. Fluoroquinolones are indicated for infections acquired outside the United States or if the organisms are resistant to TMP/SMZ.

T ABLE 12.4. Fluid therapy for dehydration

Degree of dehydration	Signs	Rehydration therapy[a]	Replacement of ongoing stool losses	Maintenance therapy[b]
Severe (≥10%)	Signs of moderate dehydration plus: Rapid/weak pulse or Cyanosis/cold extremities or Rapid breathing or Lethargy/coma	IV fluid (Ringer's lactate 20 ml/kg/h), until pulse and state of consciousness return to baseline, then ORS 50–100 ml/kg	ORS 10 ml/kg or $^{1}/_{2}$–1 cup for each diarrheal stool and 2 ml/kg for each episode of emesis	Breastfeeding, or half-strength lactose-containing milk/formula, or undiluted lactose-free formula, or juices
Moderate (6%–9%)	↓ Skin turgor Sunken eyes or fontanelle Very dry buccal mucous membranes	ORS, 100 ml/kg	As above	As above
Mild (3%–5%)	Watery diarrhea ↑Thirst Slightly dry buccal mucous– membranes	ORS, 50 ml/kg	As above	As above
Not Detectable (<3%)	Watery diarrhea	None required	As above	As above

[a]Administer for 4 h, then reassess. If dehydration persists, repeat until dehydration resolves.

[b]Older children and adults are advised to continue taking their usual diet.

[c]Lower sodium ORS (e.g., Pedialyte or Ricelyte, containing 40–60 mEq sodium per liter) can be used to replace ongoing fluid losses. ORS, oral rehydration solution.

From Greenberg HB, Matsui SM, Louri JS. Small intestine with common bacterial and viral pathogens. In: Yamada T, Alpers DH, Laine L, Owyang C, Powell DW, eds. Textbook of Gastroenterology, 3rd ed. Philadelphia: Lippincott Williams & Wilkins, 1999:1526.

The decision to treat patients who have *Salmonella* with antibiotics depends on the patient's age, health, and immune status. Healthy patients with mild or moderate symptoms should generally not be treated because antibiotic therapy may prolong the carrier state. However, adult patients with fever, systemic symptoms, or bloody diarrhea should be treated with a fluoroquinolone. Children aged 2 months to 12 years in whom a fluoroquinolone is contraindicated can be treated with TMP-SMZ. In

T ABLE 12.5. Antibiotic treatment for infectious diarrhea

Indications	Treatment*	
Campylobacter jejuni	Primary choices:	Ciprofloxacin (CiPro), 500 mg po bid × 5 d
		*Or norfloxacin (Noroxin), 400 mg po bid × 5 d
		Or azithromycin (Zithromax), 500 mg po qid × 3 d
	Alternative:	*Erythromycin 500 mg po qid × 5 d
Clostridium difficile	Primary choice:	Metronidazole (Flagyl), 500 mg po qid × 10–14 d
	Alternative:	Vancomycin (Vancocin), 125 mg po qid × 10–14 d
Traveler's diarrhea	Primary choice:	Ciprofloxacin, 500 mg po bid × 3 d
		Or norfloxacin, 400 mg po bid × 3 d
		Or ofloxacin (Floxin), 300 mg po bid × 3 d
		PLUS loperamide (Imodium), 4 mg, then 2 mg after each loose stool
		May substitute TMP/SMX-DS (Bactrim, Septra), po bid × 3 d for ciprofloxacin, norfloxacin, or ofloxacin
Shigella infection	Primary choice:	Ciprofloxacin, 500 mg po bid × 3 d
		Or norfloxacin, 400 mg po bid × 3 d
	Alternatives:	*TMP/SMX DS po, bid × 3 d
		Or azithromycin, 500 mg po × 1 d, then 250 mg po qid × 4 d
Entamoeba histolytica	Primary choice:	Metronidazole, 750 mg po tid × 7 d
		Diiodohydroxyquin (Yodoxin), 650 mg po tid × 21 d
Isospora belli	Primary choice:	*TMP/SMX DS (Bactrim Ds, Septra Ds), 160/800 mg po qid × 10 d, then bid × 3 d
Cyclospora cayentanensis	Primary choice:	Immunocompetent patients: TMP/SMX DS, 160/800 mg po bid × 7 d
Salmonella infection	No antimicrobial therapy if healthy, asymptomatic patients	
	If symptomatic or immunocompromised patients:	
	Primary choice:	Ciprofloxacin, 500 mg po bid × 3–7 d
		Or norfloxacin, 400 mg po bid × 3–7 d
	Alternative:	*TMP/SMX DS, 160/800 mg po bid × 3–7 d
Cryptosporidium	AIDS patients:	Paromomycin (Humatin), 500–750 mg po tid or qid

bid, twice daily; po, orally; qid, four times daily; tid, three times daily; TMP/SMX, trimethoprim and sulfa methoxazole; DS, double-strength.

*Not all these medications are FDA-approved for the infections discussed.

Adapted from Gilbert DN, Moellering RC Jr, Sande MA, eds. The Sanford guide to antimicrobial therapy, 29th ed. Hyde Park, VT: Antimicrobial Therapy, 1999:141.

addition, patients at risk for bacteremia, such as chronically ill individuals, HIV-infected patients, immunosuppressed patients, infants, and the elderly should be treated even for mild illness.

Treating patients with culture-proven *Campylobacter* infection shortens the duration of the illness if symptoms are not resolving by the time culture results are available. Erythromycin is the drug of choice, but quinolones are also effective.

Escherichia coli causes a wide spectrum of disease. Invasive *E. coli* infections with bloody diarrhea should be treated with TMP-SMZ or a quinolone antibiotic. Traveler's diarrhea is most commonly caused by toxigenic *E. coli*. Other organisms include *Shigella*, *Campylobacter*, *Salmonella*, and *Giardia*. Quinolones are the drugs of choice, although TMP-SMZ is also an acceptable treatment. Travelers to areas where infectious diarrhea is common can take a 3-day supply of ciprofloxacin (Cipro) and take the medication if they develop cramps or diarrhea. If greasy stools are present and no response to ciprofloxacin occurs, empiric treatment for a *Giardia* infection should be considered.

Clostridium difficile infections can be treated with metronidazole (Flagyl); an alternative is oral vancomycin (Vancocin).

Amoebic dysentery responds to metronidazole (750 mg orally three times daily for 10 days) for treatment of the trophozoites, and diiodohydroxyquin (Yodoxin) for 21 days to eliminate cysts. *Giardia* is treated with metronidazole (250 mg three times a day for 7 days) or quinacrine (Atabrine) (100 mg three times a day for 7 days).

Symptoms related to staphylococcal or clostridium food poisoning usually resolve within 24 hours. Treatment is supportive.

Consider empiric treatment in several situations, for instance, for travelers with acute diarrhea, as previously described. Patients with evidence of blood or leukocytes in their stool, suggesting bacterial infection, may warrant empiric treatment. Patients with persistent symptoms for 2 weeks or longer and suspected *Giardia* infection also benefit from a therapeutic trial of metronidazole. Acute persistent diarrhea in immunocompromised patients may improve from an empiric 10-day trial of a quinolone.

Several preparations are available for symptomatic treatment. Absorptive preparations containing kaolin and pectate (Kaopectate) are available over the counter. These products absorb water and, theoretically, make stools more formed. However, despite wide use, their efficacy is uncertain.

Bismuth subsalicylate (Pepto-Bismol) in doses in excess of those recommended on the label are sometimes effective. The antidiarrheal effect is through its antisecretory salicylate. The preparation may have some antibacterial activity which may explain its value as a prophylactic agent in traveler's diarrhea.

The antimotility drugs, such as loperamide (Imodium), are the drugs of choice for most nonspecific therapy. These medications slow gut motility, facilitating intestinal absorption. Loperamide is generally recommended because of its safety and ability to reduce stool number by 80%. Diphenoxylate (Lomotil) is less expensive but possesses central opiate activity that could be life-threatening if taken in overdose. Also, atropine is added to the drug, which can lead to anticholinergic side effects without adding antidiarrheal effects. The antimotility drugs should not be used in febrile patients with dysentery. However, most clinicians will use these medications concomitantly with antimicrobial therapy in nondysenteric forms of diarrhea. These medications are described in greater detail in Chapter 13, *Chronic Diarrhea*.

Octreotide (Sandostatin) is a drug that is sometimes used for patients with HIV-associated diarrhea that is unresponsive to usual treatment. Its cost and inconvenience (no oral form) make it a drug of last resort.

T ABLE 12.6. Advice to patients for avoiding traveler's diarrhea

Avoid	Instead choose
Water	Purified water
Ice	Carbonated drinks
Salads	Steaming hot foods and beverages
Raw vegetables	Peeled fruits
Dried foods	

FOLLOW-UP

Monitor patients with an initial presentation of mild to moderate illness to ensure that symptoms improve within 48 to 72 hours. Patients with persistent diarrhea, particularly those with HIV or who are immunosuppressed, need careful follow-up. Patients with documented intestinal amebiasis, *Salmonella*, or *Shigella* infections, need follow-up cultures to document clearing the infection. Patients whose occupation places them at risk for transmitting illness to others (e.g., food handlers) should not return to work until cultures are negative.

PATIENT EDUCATION

Education about oral rehydration and diet is important. The type of foods described are easy to take and should be adequate for therapy. After an episode of acute diarrhea, many experts recommend eliminating milk and milk products for approximately 1 week. Patients should be instructed about perianal hygiene that can ameliorate the discomfort that can accompany severe diarrhea. Sitz baths or washing with warm water using cotton may be better tolerated than toilet paper. Witch hazel-impregnated products (TUCKS) often provide relief of itching and burning.

Individuals traveling to foreign countries should be advised to avoid drinking local water and eating foods that may be contaminated (Table 12.6).

SUGGESTED READING

Ansdell VE, Ericsson CD. Prevention and empiric treatment of traveler's diarrhea. *Med Clin North Am* 1999;83:945–971.

Aranda-Michel J, Giannella RA. Acute diarrhea: a practical review. *Am Fam Physician* 1999;106:670–676.

Fekety R. Guidelines for the diagnoses and management of *Clostridium difficile*-associated diarrhea and colitis. *Am J Gastroenterol* 1997;92:739–750.

Kroser JA, Metz DC. Evaluation of the adult patient with diarrhea. *Prim Care* 1996;23: 629–647.

CHAPTER 13

Chronic Diarrhea

Martin S. Lipsky

DEFINITION

Patients can refer to any change in stool pattern as diarrhea, but diarrhea is defined as an increase in stool weight to more than 200 g/d. Fecal urgency, cramping, and loose or watery stools often accompany the increase in stool weight. Chronic diarrhea is a recurrent condition that persists for more than 3 weeks.

CLINICAL MANIFESTATIONS

The first step in the evaluation of chronic diarrhea is to confirm by history or stool collection that a patient has significant diarrhea. Once confirmed, a careful history may suggest the diagnosis or direct the workup. Table 13.1 lists the key elements of the history.

Age. The most common cause of chronic diarrhea in children of all ages is infection. Chronic diarrhea in infants aged less than 3 months suggests disaccharide deficiency, cow's milk intolerance, cystic fibrosis, or an immunodeficiency state. Chronic diarrhea in the age range from toddler to adolescent suggests celiac disease, inflammatory bowel disease (IBD), or late-onset primary lactose deficiency. A thriving toddler who is cheerful despite having diarrhea is most consistent with nonspecific diarrhea of childhood.

Character of the stool. Voluminous diarrhea suggests either malabsorption or a secretory diarrhea. Greasy, foul-smelling stools that are difficult to flush point to malabsorption. Blood or pus in the stool raises the possibility of neoplasm or IBD. Mucus indicates inflammation or irritable bowel syndrome (IBS).

Timing of the bowel movements. Nocturnal diarrhea identifies patients likely to have organic disease. Secretory diarrheas usually have no relationship to meals, whereas in patients with osmotic diarrhea (e.g., lactose deficiency) diarrhea decreases with fasting. Patients with dumping syndrome, most commonly associated with a surgical history of vagotomy and pyloroplasty, have diarrhea triggered by meals. Passing several small stools shortly after awakening is most consistent with IBS.

Duration of symptoms. Classifying diarrhea as either acute (< 3 weeks) or chronic is useful because most viral causes and transient dietary-induced diarrhea resolve within a period of 2 to 3 weeks. Small volume diarrhea alternating with constipation is most consistent with IBS, diverticulosis, or less so, colon cancer.

Associated intestinal symptoms. Lower abdominal cramping associated with fecal urgency and relieved with defecation suggests a colonic disorder. Cramping and periumbilical pains are commonly seen in patients with IBS. Tenesmus, the sensation of incomplete rectal emptying, suggests rectal involvement. Conditions associated with tenesmus include proctitis from infectious disease or IBD, anorectal fissures, and anorectal carcinoma.

Fever. Fever is not present in most diseases causing chronic diarrhea. Its presence suggests the possibility of inflammatory disease, lymphoma, human immunodeficiency virus (HIV)-associated diarrheal illness, and amebiasis.

T ABLE 13.1. Important elements to evaluate in patients with diarrhea

Character of the stool
Timing of bowel movements
Duration of symptoms
Associated intestinal symptoms
Fever
Weight loss
Medications
Past surgical and medical history
Dietary history
Travel history

Weight loss is associated with malabsorption, IBD, or malignancy. It is uncommon in IBS or lactose intolerance.

Medications. Antibiotic use can be associated with diarrhea; they can cause abdominal pain, fever, and profuse watery stools. Table 13.2 lists medications associated with diarrhea.

Surgical history. Surgery to treat peptic ulcer disease can result in diarrhea associated with rapid dumping of intestinal contents into the small bowel. Gastrointestinal surgery can also cause diarrhea by creating blind loops or short bowel syndrome. Cholecystectomy can lead to diarrhea, possibly induced by bile salts.

Medical history. Diarrhea, particularly nocturnal, is associated with an autonomic diabetic neuropathy. Scleroderma can cause small bowel dysfunction and diarrhea. Previous pelvic or abdominal radiation can cause a radiation enterocolitis that can present months to years after treatment.

Dietary history. Diarrhea can be caused by milk or milk products in patients with lactose deficiency or by gluten-containing foods in patients with celiac sprue. Sorbitol or fructose-sweetened foods can cause osmotic diarrhea. In general, osmotic diarrhea stops when the patient fasts or stops ingesting the absorbable solute. Heavy alcohol consumption can also lead to diarrhea.

T ABLE 13.2. Common drugs associated with diarrhea

Alcohol
Antacids containing magnesium
Antibiotics
Colchicine
Guanethidine (Ismelin)
Lactulose
Laxatives
Loop diuretics
Propranolol (Inderal)
Quinidine
Theophylline
Thyroxine

T ABLE 13.3.   Associated symptoms that may give clues to the cause of diarrhea

Clinical findings	Diagnoses to be considered
Arthritis	Ulcerative colitis, Crohn's disease, Whipple's disease
Liver disease	Ulcerative colitis, Crohn's disease, bowel malignancy with metastases to liver
Fever	Ulcerative colitis, Crohn's disease, amoebiasis, lymphoma, tuberculosis
Marked weight loss	Malabsorption, inflammatory bowel disease, cancer, thyrotoxicosis
Eosinophilia	Eosinophilic gastroenteritis, parasitic disease
Lymphadenopathy	Lymphoma, Whipple's disease, AIDS
Neuropathy	Diabetic diarrhea, amyloidosis
Postural hypotension	Diabetic diarrhea, Addison's disease, idiopathic orthostatic hypotension
Flushing	Malignant carcinoid syndrome, pancreatic cholera
Proteinuria	Amyloidosis
Perianal disease or abdominal mass in the right lower quadrant	Crohn's disease
Purpura	Celiac disease
Peptic ulcer	Zollinger-Ellison syndrome, antacid therapy, gastrocolic fistula
After cholecystectomy	Bile acid malabsorption
After gastrectomy	Dumping syndrome
Frequent infections	Immunoglobulin deficiency, AIDS
Immunodeficiency	Giardiasis, nodular lymphoid hyperplasia, celiac sprue, AIDS
Hyperpigmentation	Whipple's disease, celiac disease, Addison's disease
Good response to antibiotics	Bacterial overgrowth in small intestines

AIDS, acquired immune deficiency syndrome.

Travel history. Most diarrheal illnesses associated with travel are acute; however, amebiasis and giardiasis can lead to chronic diarrhea.

Associated extraintestinal symptoms can also provide clues to the cause of diarrhea. Flushing or wheezing suggests carcinoid syndrome. Arthritis, uveitis, and pyoderma gangrenosum are sometimes seen in patients with IBD. Table 13.3 lists other associated symptoms that offer clues to the cause of diarrhea.

Physical examination is useful for determining how urgently an evaluation is needed. Patients who appear toxic or dehydrated (e.g., orthostatic, poor skin turgor) may need hospitalization for rehydration, evaluation, and treatment. Physical examination is less helpful than the history in determining a diagnosis. A right lower quadrant mass and anorectal fissure are consistent with Crohn's disease. Pyoderma gangrenosum, erythema nodosum, and uveitis are also suggestive of inflammatory bowel disorders. Hyperpigmentation suggests Addison's or Whipple's disease. A rectal mass may indicate the presence of a villous adenoma.

RISK FACTORS

Asian patients are at the greatest risk for **lactose intolerance**, whereas Northern Europeans have the lowest incidence. Table 13.4 gives the prevalence of lactase deficiency in different populations.

TABLE 13.4. Lactose deficiency

Population	Prevalence (%)
Northern European	5–15
African Black	85–100
American Black	45–80
American Caucasian	10–25
Asian	90–100
Mediterranean	60–85

Lactose-containing foods can also contribute to diarrhea in patients with an underlying bowel conditions.

Chronic alcohol abuse can place patients at risk for diarrhea by its potential for causing damage to the small bowel and to the pancreas.

Recent travel to an area endemic for *Giardiasis* organisms or *Entamoeba histolytica* places patients at risk for these infections.

Previous abdominal surgery that produces a blind loop predisposes patients to bacterial over-growth and diarrhea.

Patients with **eating disorders** are more likely to abuse laxatives.

Sexual promiscuity, homosexuality, or intravenous drug use should raise suspicions of HIV-related infections.

Impaired immunity is a risk for intestinal infections, particularly protozoal infections such as *Giardia* or cryptosporidiosis.

EPIDEMIOLOGY

In an outpatient primary care setting, the most common causes of chronic diarrhea are IBS, IBD, lactose intolerance, diarrhea secondary to medications, and chronic or relapsing gastrointestinal infections (e.g., giardiasis, amebiasis, and *Clostridium difficile*).

Irritable bowel syndrome accounts for approximately half of the gastrointestinal complaints seen by physicians. Symptoms compatible with IBS occur in as many as 10% to 20% of adults, although only approximately one-third to one-half of these patients seek medical attention. The disorder most commonly affects young or middle-aged adults, with a 2:1 female:male ratio. A history of stress, emotional conflict, or anxiety is common in patients with IBS.

Inflammatory bowel disease. Age-specific incidence rates for both ulcerative colitis and Crohn's disease exhibit a bimodal distribution. The largest peak occurs in the third decade of life and a smaller peak in the sixth decade. The incidence rate for Crohn's disease is approximately 20% higher in women, whereas the incidence rate of ulcerative colitis is approximately 20% higher in men. Jewish people also tend to have higher rates of IBD.

Lactose intolerance, which affects more than half of the world's population, is categorized as (a) congenital, (b) primary with delayed onset, or (c) secondary. The most common is delayed onset, where the level of lactase decreases to 5% to 10% of the amount seen at birth. A secondary deficiency occurs when enzyme activity decreases as a result of diffuse intestinal insult, such as seen in *Giardia* infections or Crohn's disease.

Giardiasis is the most common protozoal infection worldwide. Although far more prevalent in underdeveloped countries, its prevalence is still 2% to 5% in developed countries.

Amebiasis is more commonly seen in underdeveloped countries where sanitation is poor.

Clostridium difficile is associated with the use of antibiotics and infection can occur up to 8 weeks after antibiotic use. It can occur with any antibiotic but is more commonly seen with broad-spectrum antibiotics.

PATHOPHYSIOLOGY

Fluid balance in the gastrointestinal system represents a dynamic flux between absorption and secretion. Conditions that either increase fluid secretion or decrease absorption lead to diarrhea. Inflammation, hormones, or enterotoxins can trigger increased fluid secretion. A functional or anatomic decrease in the absorptive capacity of the bowel can cause diarrhea. Altered bowel motility can impair absorption, either by decreasing the contact time of intestinal contents with the bowel mucosa or by preventing the effective mixing of intestinal contents. Osmotically active solutes (e.g., sorbitol) that retain fluid in the intestinal lumen can also increase stool volume. Although the basic mechanisms of diarrhea are straightforward, more than one mechanism may cause diarrhea in a single patient. For example, in a patient with Crohn's disease, an abnormal ileum may cause decreased fluid absorption as well as increased secretion as a result of diffuse inflammation.

DIFFERENTIAL DIAGNOSIS

Table 13.5 lists the extensive differential diagnoses for chronic diarrhea. The workup for diarrhea should be individualized. A thorough history reviewing past medical illnesses and surgeries, travel history, diet history, and medications will give ample clues to the diagnosis. For patients whose history and physical suggest a benign cause and have no indication suggestive of serious disease, a minimal workup may be needed. For example, patients with suspected lactose intolerance who respond to a lactose-free diet need no further testing. Similarly, a patient with diarrhea who is taking an antacid and responds to decreasing or stopping the medication needs no further evaluation. Up to 4% of causes of chronic diarrhea are the result of medication and food additives such as sorbitol.

If a diagnosis is not readily apparent from the history and physical examination, **an initial workup** may consist of a complete blood cell count, erythrocyte sedimentation rate, and stool studies. For a patient with loose stools, associated left lower quadrant pain, or bloody diarrhea, early sigmoidoscopy examination is often helpful. Stool studies consist of examining the stool for ova and parasites, occult blood, and a smear for leukocytes. At least three stools should be checked for *Giardia* organisms because stool excretion can be intermittent.

If a Wright's or Gram's stain reveals large numbers of leukocytes, consider IBD or an infection. For patients with suspected malabsorption, their stools can be qualitatively tested for fat using a Sudan fat stain. Blood in the stool increases the likelihood for neoplasm or inflammatory disease. In suspected laxative abuse, alkalinizing the stool can detect phenolphthalein by turning the stool a pinkish color. An assay for *C. difficile* toxin is helpful in patients with diarrhea and recent antibiotic exposure.

Blood tests may be useful, but are rarely diagnostic. A complete blood count can detect patients with an anemia or leukocytosis. Serum amylase can be elevated in

T ABLE 13.5. Possible underlying causes of chronic diarrhea

IDIOPATHIC SECRETORY DIARRHEA
Collagenous colitis
Microscopic colitis

INFECTIONS
Amoebiasis
Giardiasis
Opportunistic infections associated with immunodeficiency states such as acquired immunodeficiency syndrome

TUMORS
Colon cancer
Endocrine tumor, such as carcinoid and gastrinoma
Intestinal lymphoma
Medullary carcinoma of the thyroid
Pancreatic carcinoma
Villous adenoma

LACTOSE INTOLERANCE
Malabsorption
Bacterial overgrowth
Bile-salt deficiency
Pancreatic insufficiency
Small bowel diseases, such as celiac sprue, short bowel syndrome, Whipple's disease

MECHANICAL FACTORS
Fecal impaction
Postsurgical syndromes

METABOLIC DISORDERS
Addison's disease
Diabetes
Hyperthyroidism

pancreatic disease and abnormal liver function tests may indicate hepatobiliary dysfunction. Serum calcium and glucose may be elevated in metabolic conditions associated with diarrhea. Serum electrolytes can detect abnormalities associated with fluid losses. Additional specialized blood testing may be appropriate, based on history and physical. For example, gastrin levels are indicated in patients with severe peptic ulcer disease and watery diarrhea. Urinary level of 5-hydroxyindoleacetic acid is helpful to screen for carcinoid in patients with undiagnosed diarrhea and flushing. An antigliadin antibody is a useful test for patients with suspected celiac sprue.

Sigmoidoscopy should be considered when blood or leukocytes are found in the stool. This procedure can detect ulcerations, friability, and masses. If ulcerations are seen and amebiasis is suspected, a mucosal smear should be examined for

T ABLE 13.6. Findings suggestive of organic disease

New onset of symptoms in patients >40 y
Nocturnal symptoms
Progressive course
Weight loss
Rectal fissures
Anemia
Elevated erythrocyte sedimentation rate
Greasy stools that are difficult to flush

the presence of amoeba. Suspected IBD may be confirmed by biopsy. Biopsy may also detect amyloidosis, Whipple's disease, microscopic colitis, and collageneous colitis.

Radiologic examinations may be useful in demonstrating anatomic abnormalities (e.g., blind loops, fistulas, and tumors). A flat plate to check for pancreatic calcifications suggests the presence of pancreatic insufficiency. Barium studies can help determine the extent and presence of mucosal diseases.

The diagnosis of IBS is usually made clinically. Criteria suggesting IBS include (a) continuous or recurrent symptoms over several months associated with abdominal pain that is relieved by defecation or associated with a change in frequency or consistency of stool, or (b) a varied pattern of disturbed defecation occurring 25% of the time and consisting of two or more of the following: change in frequency and consistency of stool, straining, urgency, passage of mucus, bloating, or a feeling of incomplete evacuation. Table 13.6 lists factors that increase the likelihood for underlying organic disease history. A cost-effective method of evaluating patients with IBS includes a careful history and physical examination and a limited workup to exclude the possibility of serious disease.

REFERRAL

Referral to a gastroenterologist for a more detailed evaluation is helpful in patients whose diagnosis remains uncertain after the initial workup. The most common organic causes found at this stage of workup are IBD (including microscopic and collagenous colitis) and IBS. In addition, surreptitious laxative abuse accounts for 3.5% to 7% of these obscure cases and should be excluded before subjecting the patient to an extensive evaluation.

Inpatient evaluation is sometimes needed because of persistent troublesome diarrhea. Evaluation of these patients includes quantitative stool fat analysis, stool electrolytes, and monitoring the patient's response to fasting. Quantitative stool fat analysis requires collecting stools for 72 hours while the patient is on a prescribed diet. This test is indicated when a qualitative study (e.g., Sudan stain) is positive and routinely in patients with persistent diarrhea of unknown origin. Diarrhea that responds to fasting and also has an osmotic gap in stool electrolytes is usually the result of laxative abuse, unabsorbed carbohydrates, or bile acid secretion. Table 13.7 classifies diarrhea by the level of response to diet.

Patients with severe underlying causes for diarrhea (e.g., neoplasm or IBD) should generally be referred to a specialist expert in managing these conditions.

T ABLE 13.7. Diarrhea disorders and response to fasting

DECREASE WITH FASTING

Bile acid diarrhea
  Postcholecystectomy
  Postileac resection
Malabsorption
Osmotic diarrhea
  Carbohydrate malabsorption
    Osmotically active laxatives (i.e., Milk of Magnesia)
Food allergies

NONRESPONSE TO FASTING

Stimulant laxative abuse
Inflammatory bowel disease
Celiac sprue
Intestinal lymphoma
Neuroendocrine diseases
Zollinger-Ellison's syndrome
Carcinoid disease
Villous adenoma
Chronic infections
Hyperthyroidism
Bacterial overgrowth

MANAGEMENT

Management depends on the underlying causes of the diarrhea. Occasionally, an empirical trial is helpful if a specific diagnosis is suspected. For example, pancreatic enzymes might be tried when pancreatic insufficiency is suspected. *Giardia* infection is commonly missed on stool examinations and a treatment trial of metronidazole may be warranted in patients with chronic diarrhea and a history of travel to an endemic area. Trials of lactose-free or gluten-free diets are also helpful on occasion.

Lactose intolerance. Typically, a lactose-intolerant individual will respond to 1 to 2 weeks of a lactose-free diet. Individuals may eat dairy products pretreated with lactase. Lactase capsules can be taken orally before consuming diary products or lactase drops can be added to milk.

Irritable bowel syndrome. No test is diagnostic for IBS. Similarly, no one treatment is always successful. Patients whose predominant symptom is diarrhea may find relief with an antidiarrheal medication, such as loperamide (Imodium), 2 to 4 mg up to four times daily, or diphenoxylate hydrochloride with atropine (Lomotil), 10 to 20 mg up to four times a day. Antispasmotics, such as dicyclomine (Bentyl), 10 to 20 mg before meals, may benefit patients with associated abdominal cramping and pain. A high-fiber diet is most appropriate for IBS patients who predominantly have constipation but can also be helpful in patients with diarrhea that alternates with constipation. A fiber supplement (e.g., psyllium) may be beneficial in selected patients. Psyllium should be started slowly (at 1 tsp/d) and increased weekly as needed up to three times a day. In some patients, stress management and counseling may be beneficial.

Some patients, particularly those with underlying depression or sleep disturbances, may benefit from a tricyclic antidepressant.

Management goals for patients with **inflammatory bowel disease** are to control active disease, maintain remission, detect complications, and refer to surgery, when appropriate. In addition to medications, the patient's nutritional status and psychological well-being need to be addressed. Most patients should be comanaged with a gastroenterologist experienced in managing IBD.

Ulcerative colitis typically follows a relapsing course. Sulfasalazine (Azulfidine) or one of the newer products, such as mesalamine (Asacol, Pentasa), that delivers 5-aminosalicylic acid to the colonic mucosa is recommended as initial therapy for mild to moderate disease and for maintaining remission (Table 13.8). Nausea, vomiting, and headache are common side effects of sulfasalazine. Occasionally, some patients may have a hypersensitivity reaction, such as a rash and fever. Because sulfasalazine is a sulfa drug, patients with a sulfa allergy should use mesalamine. Table 13.9 lists treatments for IBD.

Systemic steroids should be used in patients with moderate to extensive ulcerative colitis. Initial treatment is prednisone (40 to 60 mg daily), which can be tapered once symptoms are controlled. Typically, steroids are tapered by 5 to 10 mg a week until the dosage is 15 to 20 mg daily. The dosage is then tapered to 2.5 to 5 mg until the drug is discontinued. Patients with mild to moderate disease limited to the distal colon may benefit from mesalamine (Rowasa) or hydrocortisone enemas. Patients requiring high-

T ABLE 13.8. Inflammatory bowel disease

Disorder	Management
Ulcerative proctitis	5-ASA or corticosteroid enemas
Ulcerative colitis—mild to moderate disease	Oral 5-ASA
	Add oral steroid if needed
	Consider 5-ASA prophylaxis
Ulcerative colitis—moderate to severe	Oral steroids with or without 5-ASA
	IV steroids for severe disease
	Consider 5-ASA prophylaxis
	Referral for immunosuppresent therapy
Crohn's disease with perianal disease	Metronidazole
	Surgical evaluation if drainage needed
Mild Crohn's disease	5-ASA or metronidazole
	Add steroids if needed
	Taper therapy and follow patient
	Consider 5-ASA prophylaxis for recurrent disease
Moderate Crohn's disease	Prednisone with or without 5-ASA
	IV steroids and consider TPN if treatment fails
Severe Crohn's disease	IV steroids
	TPN
	Metronidazole

5-ASA, 5-aminosalicylic acid, mesalamine; IV, intravenous; TPN, total parenteral nutrition.

T ABLE 13.9. Medications for inflammatory bowel disease

Medication	Dosage range	Side effects
Sulfasalazine (Azulfidine)	2–4 g daily in divided doses Initially, 1–2 g after meals; increased gradually to 3–4 g if needed; maintenance dose is usually 2 g	Anorexia, GI upset, head- aches, hypersensitivity reactions, anemia
Olsalazine (Dipentum)	1–3 g/d, starting dose; 500 mg twice daily	Diarrhea, rash
Mesalamine (Pentasa)	2–4 g/d, starting with 1 g/d	GI upset, headache, rash
Mesalamine (Asacol)	1.6–4.8 g daily, starting dose 800 mg thrice daily for 6 wk; maintenance 800 mg twice daily	GI upset

GI, gastrointestinal.

dose steroids may benefit from steroid-sparing immunosuppressant therapy with 6-mer-captopurine or azathioprine (Imuran). Although immunosupressant agents have significant side effects, they are safer and better tolerated than long-term corticosteroid treatment. Surgery should be considered in patients with high-grade dysplasia, carcinoma, or intractable symptoms on maximal medical therapy. Symptomatic care with loperamide or similar agents may be helpful. These medications should be used with caution in acutely ill patients to avoid precipitating toxic megacolon.

Maintaining adequate nutrition is critical in **Crohn's disease**. Patients with cramps and diarrhea may benefit from reduced fiber diets and nutritional supplements, such as Ensure or Isocal. Sulfasalazine or equivalent drugs are of modest benefit in inducing remission. Although it has been felt that 5-aminosalicylic acid products were not useful in maintaining remission, many gastroenterologists now advise maintenance treatment. Corticosteroids are useful in acutely ill patients or in those who do not respond to sulfasalazine. As acute disease improves, steroids should be tapered. Chronic steroid therapy is not indicated in Crohn's disease. Metronidazole is also effective in patients with acute Crohn's disease, especially in patients who have perianal manifestations. Surgery is indicated in patients who have intractable symptoms, perforation, obstruction, or severe bleeding.

Giardiasis is treated with metronidazole (250 mg three times daily for 7 to 10 days). Retreatment is sometimes necessary. Quinacrine (100 mg three times daily) is an alternative medication.

Chronic pancreatic disease causing steatorrhea usually responds to pancreatic enzymes and a low fiber diet.

Bile salt diarrhea may respond to cholesteramine, which binds the irritative bile salts. Doses in the range of 4 to 8 g daily are usually effective.

Chronic diarrhea of uncertain origin. For patients who remain undiagnosed after an exhaustive workup, treating for IBS is reasonable. Other nonspecific medications include antimotility agents such as loperamide and diphenoxylate. Loperamide (Imodium) is given initially at 4 mg then 2 mg after each loose stool with a maximum dosage of 8 mg/d for 2 days. Diphenoxylate plus atropne (Lomotil) is given as two pills up to four times a day, as needed, for diarrhea.

Amebiasis is treated with metronidazole (750 mg three times daily for 10 days), plus a second drug (e.g., diidohydroxyquin, 600 mg three times daily for 20 days) to treat amoebic cysts.

FOLLOW-UP

Patients with **irritable bowel syndrome** should be monitored periodically. Evidence of new symptoms or an indication of organic disease merits reevaluation.

Patients with **inflammatory bowel disease** should be monitored with attention to bowel frequency, rectal bleeding, general well-being, abdominal pain, and side effects from medications. If new symptoms develop, checking a complete blood cell count and erythrocyte sedimentation rate is helpful. Periodic assessment of renal and liver function is also recommended. Patients with ulcerative colitis have an increased risk of colon cancer. The risk of malignancy is related to the extent of the disease and not to its activity. Colonoscopic surveillance is also recommended every 3 years for patients with pancolitis of more than 10 years' duration.

PATIENT EDUCATION

Ulcerative colitis patients should be instructed about their increased risk for colon cancer and the need for follow-up.

Travelers should avoid eating raw fruits and vegetables in foreign countries. Using bottled water, boiled water, or treated tap water is helpful in avoiding infection.

Patients with lactose intolerance should be instructed that the judicious use of enzyme products should allow them to ingest milk or milk products with minimal symptoms.

Patient education is essential for managing **patients with IBS** effectively. The basic elements include (a) addressing patient fears because many feel something is seriously wrong with their bowels, (b) providing a diagnosis, and (c) explaining the pathophysiologic mechanism of altered motility. Educating patients that stress may trigger symptoms may help them to cope better with these symptoms.

SUGGESTED READING

Baker EH, Sandle GI. Complications of laxative abuse. *Annu Rev Med* 1996;47: 127–134.

Botoman VA, Bonner GF, Botoman DA. Management of inflammatory bowel disease. *Am Fam Physician* 1998;57:57–72.

Farthing MJ. Giardiases. *Gastroenterol Clin North Am* 1996;25:493–515.

Leung AK, Robson WL. Evaluating the child with chronic diarrhea. *Am Fam Physician* 1996;53:635–643.

Lipsky MS, Adelman M. Chronic diarrhea. *Am Fam Physician* 1993;49:1607–1612.

CHAPTER 14

Nausea and Vomiting

Martin S. Lipsky

DEFINITION

Nausea is the sensation of having to vomit and often precedes or accompanies vomiting. Vomiting, which can either be voluntary or involuntary, is the forceful expulsion of gastric contents through the mouth. It is often accompanied by autonomic responses such as sweating, dizziness, and pallor. Anorexia is loss of appetite and differs from nausea and vomiting because patients with nausea and vomiting may still experience the urge to eat. Vomiting should also be distinguished from regurgitation. Regurgitation is when gastric or esophageal contents are returned to the mouth without the autonomic and motor responses. Regurgitation suggests gastroesophageal reflux or esophageal obstruction.

CLINICAL MANIFESTATIONS

Nausea and vomiting are common manifestations of many organic and functional disorders. A thorough history is helpful in sorting out the many causes of nausea and vomiting. Characterizing the duration, timing, frequency, and type of vomiting also helps to identify the cause.

Acute symptoms lasting less than 1 week suggest an infection, intoxication, drug effect, visceral disease, or a metabolic abnormality. **Early morning nausea and vomiting** is more typical of metabolic causes such as uremia and adrenal insufficiency or pregnancy. Nausea and vomiting symptoms triggered by eating suggest acute gastritis, peptic ulcer disease, esophageal or gastric outlet obstruction, or psychogenic factors. Vomiting several hours after eating is more consistent with gastric retention from outflow obstruction, atony from diabetic gastroparesis, anticholinergic drug use, or gastric malignancy.

Characterizing the vomitus can be helpful. **Bile**, which is commonly present with prolonged vomiting from any cause, indicates an open pyloric channel. Projectile vomiting in infants may indicate pyloric stenosis. **Feculent vomitus** is seen in patients with lower intestinal obstruction or gastrocolic fistula. **Bloody** or **coffee-ground** emesis indicates bleeding from the esophagus, stomach, or duodenum.

A careful **medication history** is indicated. Table 14.1 lists medications commonly associated with nausea and vomiting. Most cancer chemotherapeutic agents and radiation therapy can cause nausea and vomiting. Other drugs commonly associated with nausea and vomiting include opiates, anticholinergics, and erythromycin. Nausea and vomiting can also indicate toxic levels of medications. Digitalis and theophylline are among the most common drugs causing serious drug toxicity.

Nausea and vomiting accompanied by fever, watery diarrhea, and abdominal cramps is typical for viral gastroenteritis. Food poisoning from preformed toxins usually results in vomiting within 6 hours after eating the offending substance and usually resolves in 24 to 48 hours. **Abdominal pain** may indicate a surgical emergency, such as appendicitis or cholecystitis. Abdominal cramps can be caused by

TABLE 14.1. Common medications associated with nausea and vomiting

Antibiotics, especially erythromycin and metronidazole
Opiates
Nonsteroidal antiinflammatory drugs
Estrogen (e.g., birth control pills)
Digitalis
Chemotherapeutic agents
Theophylline

infection or early obstruction. Severe pain lacking cramplike qualities can be the result of peritoneal irritation or late obstruction. Visceral pain syndromes seen with myocardial infarction, pancreatitis, renal colic, and biliary colic commonly cause acute nausea.

Vertigo suggests an acute vestibular cause such as motion sickness or acute labyrinthitis. Recurrent vertigo, tinnitus, and vomiting are consistent with Ménière's disease, whereas headache and other neurologic symptoms suggest a central nervous system (CNS) cause. Projectile vomiting without nausea occurs with CNS diseases that cause increased intracranial pressure. Rarely, neurologic emergencies (e.g., cerebellar hemorrhage or meningitis) present with vomiting as the predominant symptom.

Persistent nausea and vomiting without an underlying cause suggested by history and physical is most commonly related to structural lesions affecting the upper gastrointestinal (GI) tract (e.g., peptic ulcer disease or gastric outlet syndrome).

The **medical and surgical histories** often suggest possible causes. Diabetic ketoacidosis should always be considered in diabetic patients with nausea and vomiting. Coronary artery disease or renal insufficiency raises the possibility that nausea and vomiting is caused by one of these conditions. Previous abdominal surgery may rule out causes such as appendicitis, but it increases the risk of intestinal obstruction.

PHYSICAL EXAMINATION

The physical examination should include assessment of general appearance, vital signs, and volume status. An **abdominal examination** can provide clues to the underlying pathology, particularly in patients with abdominal pain. Local tenderness may suggest a specific cause (e.g., cholecystitis, peptic ulcer disease, or pancreatitis). Tenderness with guarding and rebound tenderness occurs with peritoneal or visceral disease. With auscultation, high-pitched bowel sounds are consistent with an early obstruction, whereas decreased or absent bowel sounds occur with a late obstruction, ileus, or peritonitis. A succussion splash is consistent with gastric outlet obstruction. An **enlarged, tender liver** suggests hepatitis.

Breast tenderness or **uterine enlargement** suggests pregnancy. The nausea and vomiting of labyrinthine disorders such as Ménière's disease, benign positional vertigo, and vestibular neuronitis are frequently positional. It is important to perform a neurologic examination to look for signs of a CNS cause: a stiff neck for meningitis, papilledema for increased intracranial pressure, or ataxia in cerebellar hemorrhage.

RISK FACTORS

Very young or elderly patients and individuals with illnesses that affect fluid balance, such as renal insufficiency, have an increased risk for complications from vomiting.

Patients with underlying disorders such as coronary artery disease, diabetes, alcoholism, cancer, and liver disease are at risk for developing nausea and vomiting from either the disease itself or from a complication induced by these conditions. Individuals with endocrine disorders (e.g., hyperthyroidism, hyperparathyroidism, or adrenal insufficiency) are also at risk for nausea and vomiting.

Of pregnant women, 80% experience nausea, which resolves in half of affected women by the second trimester. Hyperemesis gravidarum develops in 0.3% of women and without treatment can produce rapid fluid shifts and dehydration that can threaten fetal viability.

Patients taking new medications are at risk for developing nausea and vomiting. Drug and alcohol use are risk factors for hepatitis, early morning "dry heaves," and withdrawal syndromes in which gastrointestinal upset may be the predominant symptom. Vomiting is often a component of eating disorders such as anorexia nervosa or bulimia, which can affect 5% to 10% of young women.

EPIDEMIOLOGY

Nausea and vomiting comprise a common presenting complaint for family physicians, ranking among the most common reasons for an office visit. In most instances, the symptoms are caused by a self-limited illness (e.g., viral gastroenteritis). Young women are more likely to have a psychogenic cause for recurrent vomiting. Table 14.2 lists common causes of nausea and vomiting encountered in the outpatient setting.

PATHOPHYSIOLOGY

The act of vomiting is under the control of two CNS centers, the vomiting center in the medullary reticular formation and the chemoreceptor trigger zone in the floor of the fourth ventricle. Vagal nerve irritation and impulses from sympathetic efferents in the throat, heart, abdomen, and GI tract can trigger impulses to the vomiting center. Vestibular disturbances, centrally acting drugs, and metabolic abnormalities can stimulate the chemoreceptor trigger zone. Afferent nerves then carry the impulses to the vomiting center. Efferent impulses then travel to effector muscles, producing a stereotypical vomiting response that varies little regardless of cause. This response includes relaxation of the gastric fundus and the gastroesophageal sphincter, contraction of the pylorus, and reverse peristalsis in the esophagus. The glottis closes and the diaphragm and abdominal muscles contract, causing a sudden increase in intraabdominal pressure that forces the stomach contents out through the mouth.

T ABLE 14.2. Common causes of nausea and vomiting in the outpatient setting

Acute viral gastroenteritis
Food poisoning
Pregnancy
Adverse drug reaction
Labyrinthitis or motion sickness

DIFFERENTIAL DIAGNOSIS

Table 14.3 lists some conditions associated with nausea and vomiting. The list encompasses a wide range of functional and organic GI disorders and various systemic conditions. However, careful history and physical examination can often indicate the diagnosis and direct the workup. For example, a review of a patient's medications may reveal the use of an agent associated with nausea and vomiting. Fever, malaise, and myalgias suggest an infectious cause.

In patients with a 1- to 2-day history of nausea and vomiting, an apparent viral illness, and no evidence of toxicity or dehydration, further evaluation is generally indicated only if the symptoms do not resolve.

In patients with **acute nausea and vomiting** and significant abdominal pain, intraabdominal pathology is likely. The first priority is to rule out an acute surgical cause (e.g., a bowel obstruction or peritonitis). Further testing should be guided by the history and physical examination. For example, obstruction should be considered in patients with colicky abdominal pain.

Chronic nausea and vomiting are commonly related to structural lesions in the upper GI tract. Endoscopy can detect mucosal lesions, ulcer disease, or gastric outlet obstruction. If endoscopy is not diagnostic, an upper GI series may be helpful. An abdominal ultrasound or computed tomography (CT) scan is indicated if endoscopic examination suggests an extrinsic process.

Recurrent vomiting of unknown cause raises the possibility of a psychological cause. Clues to a psychological disorder are presented in Table 14.4. Early morning nausea in the absence of pregnancy or metabolic abnormalities raises the possibility of increased intracranial pressure; thus, a head CT scan should be considered in making the diagnosis.

DIAGNOSTIC STUDIES

Table 14.5 summarizes tests that may be useful for evaluating patients with nausea and vomiting. Always keep in mind that a fertile woman may be pregnant or that nausea may be drug-induced. A pregnancy test and serum drug level analysis are useful in these situations. An electrocardiogram can screen for acute myocardial infarction and underlying cardiac ischemia.

Blood tests are helpful in cases of protracted vomiting, particularly in older patients or young patients in whom electrolyte abnormalities or volume depletion is more likely. Significant volume depletion elevates the blood urea nitrogen and can cause hemoconcentration and a rise in hematocrit. A complete blood count can document subacute or chronic blood loss that may suggest underlying ulcer disease. The white blood cell count is frequently elevated in patients with infection or inflammatory disease. Liver function tests are useful when hepatitis is suspected. Occasionally, an individual with a renal stone will have nausea and vomiting as the predominant symptoms; in such cases, a urine analysis is helpful.

Imaging is indicated in selected circumstances. Plain radiographic films of the abdomen can help rule out an acute obstruction. Barium studies may demonstrate a lesion or provide indirect evidence (e.g., delayed transit or bowel dilatation) that suggests a mechanical or functional obstruction.

Endoscopy is more expensive than barium studies but provides direct visualization. It detects mucosal ulceration and also provides the opportunity to obtain tissue for diagnosing malignancy. Because endoscopy is not usually helpful for diagnosing motor dysfunction, gastric emptying studies may be needed. Gastric scintography, using radiolabeled material that is swallowed and tracked through the gut, can be helpful in identifying delayed emptying. If the diagnosis is still uncertain, some spe-

T ABLE 14.3.   Differential diagnosis of nausea and vomiting

Causes of Nausea and Vomiting Usually Associated with Abdominal Pain
  Viral gastroenteritis
  Bowel obstruction
  Cholecystitis
  Gastritis
  Pancreatitis
  Peptic ulcer disease
  Pyelonephritis
  Food poisoning
  Renal colic
Common Causes of Acute Vomiting Not Usually Associated with Abdominal Pain
  Pregnancy
  Metabolic disorders
  Drug withdrawal
  Hepatitis
  Binge drinking
  Systemic infections (especially in children)
Nausea and Vomiting in Association with Neurologic Symptoms
  Labyrinthitis
  Head trauma
  Migraine headache
  Increased intracranial pressure
  Cerebellar hemorrhage
  Meningitis
  Central nervous system neoplasm
Recurrent or Chronic Vomiting
  Psychogenic
  Metabolic disturbances (e.g., uremia)
  Peptic ulcer disease
  Gastric outlet obstruction
  Bile reflux after gastric surgery
Less Common Causes of Vomiting in the Primary Care Setting
  Myocardial infarction
  Ketoacidosis
  Addisonian crisis
  Diabetic gastroparesis
  Lactic acidosis
  Congestive heart failure
  Metastatic cancer
  Gastrointestinal neoplasm

Adapted from Evaluation of nausea and vomiting. In: Goroll AE, May LA, Mulley AG, eds. *Primary Care Medicine*, 3rd ed. Philadelphia: Lippincott-Raven, 1995:336.

T ABLE 14.4. Clues to psychogenic vomiting

Chronic emesis
Vomiting around mealtimes
Conflict-ridden social situations
Normal appetite despite nausea and vomiting
Inappropriate attitude toward symptoms
Inappropriate attitude to weight loss, if present

T ABLE 14.5. Selected tests for evaluating nausea and vomiting

Test	Diagnostic consideration
Plain films of abdomen	Obstruction, ileus
Endoscopy	Gastritis, peptic ulcer disease, pyloric channel deformity
Abdominal ultrasound	Biliary disease, peritonitis
Electrocardiograph	Myocardial infarction
Uric acid levels	Renal colic, dehydration, pyelonephritis
β–HCG level	Pregnancy
Liver function tests	Hepatitis, cholestasis
Blood urea nitrogen, creatinine	Dehydration, uremia
Glucose	Diabetic ketoacidosis, diabetic gastroparesis
Electrolytes	Ketoacidosis, adrenal insufficiency, dehydration
Amylase, lipase	Pancreatitis
Complete blood count	Appendicitis, peritonitis, or other acute infection
Digoxin level	Digitalis toxicity
Abdominal CT scan	Further evaluation of abdominal mass or biliary pathology
Head CT or MRI scans	Central nervous system pathologic condition
Stool guaiac	Ulcer disease

CT, computed tomography; HCG, human chorionic gonadotropin; MRI, magnetic resonance imaging.

cialized centers are able to perform manometry under fasting and postprandial conditions. This can provide information about neuropathic and myopathic involvement. An algorithm for evaluating dysmotility is shown in Figure 14.1.

REFERRAL

Patients with evidence of mechanical obstruction or peritonitis should be referred for hospitalization and consultation. Patients with dehydration may require intravenous fluid administration. Patients with surgical problems (e.g., suspected appendicitis and cholecystitis) causing vomiting should also be referred for evaluation. Patients with recalcitrant hyperemesis gravidarum may benefit from obstetric and dietary consultations. Patients with conditions causing increased intracranial pressure or those with acute cerebellar hemorrhage should be referred to neurology or neurosurgery. Psychogenic vomiting should be evaluated by a psychiatrist.

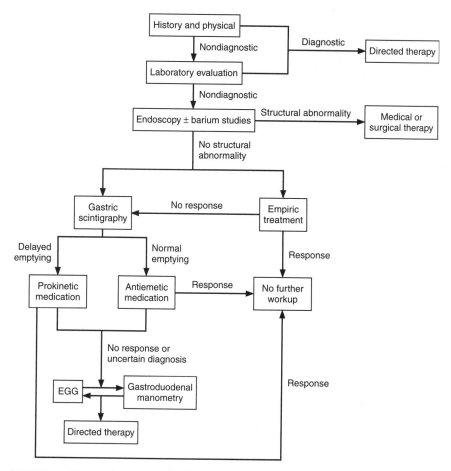

FIGURE 14.1. An algorithm for the evaluation of the patient with a presumed gastrointestinal dysmotility syndrome. (From Hasler WL. Approach to the patient with nausea and vomiting. In: Yamada T, Alpers DH, Laine L, Owyang C, Powell DW, eds. *Textbook of gastroenterology*. Philadelphia: Lippincott Williams & Wilkins; 1999:786.)

MANAGEMENT

Management should be directed at the underlying cause. If a viral infection is causing the nausea and vomiting, supportive care with fluids or electrolytes is indicated. Bacterial infections should be treated with appropriate antibiotic therapy. With no signs of underlying pathology, simple dietary measures may suffice. Mild cases can be managed with clear liquids ingested in small amounts at frequent intervals.

Nausea and vomiting resulting from a medication usually resolve by discontinuing the offending agent. If the drug is essential, nausea may be relieved by decreasing the dose, changing the timing of the dose (many drugs are better tolerated with food), or changing to another preparation. Antiemetics can also be prescribed after other causes are ruled out.

Pregnancy-associated symptoms often respond to changes in diet, eating smaller meals, placing dry crackers at the bedside to eat before getting out of bed, and avoiding foods with strong odors. Some evidence indicates that 25 mg of vitamin B_6 can alleviate nausea symptoms in pregnancy.

Medications that provide symptomatic relief are helpful for improving patient comfort and preventing complications. However, these drugs have side effects, especially in children, and are not considered completely safe for pregnant patients. Many also do not have US Food and Drug Administration indications for treating nausea and vomiting.

Antiemetic drugs are usually divided into two classes: (a) centrally acting and (b) affecting the gastrointestinal tract. Central agents work by suppressing the chemoreceptor trigger zone.

The phenothiazines are centrally acting agents that are good initial choices for controlling symptoms resulting from drugs, metabolic disorders, or gastroenteritis. Prochlorperazine (Compazine) and promethazine (Phenergan) are among the most commonly used agents. Prochlorperazine is given orally every 6 hours (5 to 10 mg) or rectally every 8 to 12 hours (25 mg). The oral dosage of promethazine is 12.5 to 25 mg every 4 to 6 hours; the rectal dose is 25 mg three times daily. Their most common side effect is sedation, but they can cause extrapyramidal side effects, especially in children.

Trimethobenzamide (Tigan) is a nonphenothiazine centrally acting drug. The dosage is 250 mg three times a day or 200 mg per rectal suppository three times a day. The oral centrally acting drugs are less effective in patients with vestibular disease. For relief of vestibular symptoms, the antihistamine meclizine (Antivert) is helpful. The average effective dose is 25 mg four times daily. Other antihistamines such as dimenhydrinate (Dramamine) or diphenhydramine (Benadryl) are also effective. All centrally acting agents and antihistamines can cause drowsiness. Caution patients regarding use of these agents when driving or operating machinery.

For patients with motility disorders or vomiting secondary to chemotherapeutic drugs, prokinetic agents that affect the GI tract may be helpful. Metoclopramide (Reglan) is an agent that acts both centrally and peripherally. The dosage is 10 mg orally or intravenously up to four times daily. Side effects include anxiety, extrapyramidal reactions (especially in children), and, rarely, tardive dyskinesia.

Cisapride (Propulsid), a benzamide derivative with prokinetic activity, is effective in improving symptoms in patients with delayed gastric emptying. Side effects include diarrhea and abdominal cramps. The dosage is 10 to 20 mg before meals and at bedtime. Numerous drug interactions have been reported with this medication and it should be used cautiously, particularly with macrolides, long-acting antihistamines, and antifungal agents (Table 14.6). At press time, Cisapride was expected to be voluntarily withdrawn from the U.S. market because of concerns about heart rhythm abnormalities.

Scopolamine, an antichoinergic medication, is used primarily for motion sickness prophylaxis. It comes as both a pill (Scopace) and a patch (Transderm-Scop). The patch is placed behind the ear and should be applied at least 4 hours before travel. Each patch provides 3 days of prophylaxis. The pill is given in a dose of 0.4 to 0.8 mg and should be started 1 hour before travel and repeated every 8 hours as needed. Scopolamine is contraindicated in patients with narrow-angle glaucoma and should be used cautiously in patients susceptible to constipation or urinary retention. Other side effects include dry mouth, blurred vision, and confusion.

Psychogenic vomiting is best managed in consultation with psychiatry. No controlled studies have examined the effectiveness of antiemetic agents in this group.

In hepatitis, nausea and vomiting may respond to phenothiazines. However, these drugs are metabolized by the liver and should be used cautiously.

The selective serotonin antagonists, ondansetron (Zofran) and granisetron (Kytril), act at the level of the CNS and GI tract. These agents are effective in chemically induced nausea and vomiting. The effectiveness of these agents may be enhanced when they are given in combination with dexamethasone (Decadron). The antiemetic agents are summarized in Table 14.7.

T ABLE 14.6.   Drugs with which Cisapride is contraindicated[a]

Macrolides	Long-acting antihistamines
Clarithromycin (Biaxin)	Astemizole (Hismanal)
Erythromycin	Class IA antiarrythmics
Antifungal Agents	Quinidine
Fluconazole (Diflucan)	Procainamide (Procanbid)
Itraconazole (Sporanox)	Miscellaneous
Antidepressants	Grapefruit juice
Tricyclics (e.g., amitriptyline)	Sparfloxacin (Zagam)
Nefazodone (Serzone)	

[a]At press time, Cisapride was expected to be voluntarily withdrawn from the U.S. market because of concerns about heart rhythm abnormalities.

T ABLE 14.7.   Characteristics of antiemetic medications

Drug class	Medications	Clinical uses	Side effects
Antihistamines	Dimenhydrinate (Dramamine)	Motion sickness	Sedation
	Meclizine (Antivert)	Labyrinthitis	Dry mouth
	Promethazine (Phenergan)	Uremia Postoperative nausea	
Antidopaminergics	Prochlorperazine (Compazine)	Extensive indications, including gastroenteritis, postoperative vomiting, migraine, medications	Sedation Anxiety Dystonic reactions Tardive dyskinesia Galactorrhea Sexual dysfunction
Prokinectic agents	Metoclopramide (Reglan)	Gastroparesis Chemotherapy-induced nausea	Extrapyramidal effects Tardive dyskinesia
	Cisapride (Propulsid)[a]	Gastroesophageal reflux Intestinal pseudoobstruction	Sedation Headache, arrythmias
Serotonin antagonists	Ondansetron (Zofran)	Chemotherapy-induced nausea	Headache, rash
	Granisetron (Kytril)	Postoperative nausea	Diarrhea
Anticholinergics	Scopolamine (Transderm Scop)	Postoperative nausea Motion sickness	Sedation Dry mouth Headache, constipation Confusion, urinary retract

[a]At press time, Cisapride was expected to be voluntarily withdrawn from the U.S. market because of concerns about heart rhythm abnormalities.

FOLLOW-UP

Recurrent emesis can cause complications such as hematemesis from esophageal tears, dehydration, aspiration pneumonia, and, rarely, esophageal rupture. Patients treated symptomatically should be monitored for adherence and the resolution of symptoms. Patients with eating disorders should be followed carefully. In addition to complications from vomiting itself, these disorders can be fatal if not aggressively treated.

PATIENT EDUCATION

Advising patients about how to manage mild nausea and vomiting can avoid unnecessary office visits. Anticipatory guidance for parents should include instruction on how to manage children with vomiting and when a doctor's appointment should be made. Individuals who are prescribed medication should be advised if nausea is a common side effect. Often, nausea can be avoided with proper instruction about how and when to take medications.

SUGGESTED READING

Friedman LS, Isselbacher KJ. Anorexia, nausea, vomiting, and indigestion. In: Wilson JD, Braunwald E, et al., eds. *Harrison's principles of internal medicine*. New York: McGraw-Hill; 1991.

Barbara G, Miglioli M. Nausea and vomiting. In: Porro GB, ed. *Gastroenterology and hepatology*. London: McGraw-Hill; 1999.

SUBJECT INDEX

Page numbers followed by f indicate figures; those followed by t indicate tables